Looking Great...

G. P. Putnam's Sons

NEW YORK

Looking Great...

Fashion Authority and Television Star Linda Dano

Shares Her Style and Beauty Secrets to

Help You Look Your Best

Linda Dano

with Anne Kyle

• *Illustrations by Barbara Griffel* •

To my mother, who taught me style,
and to my father, who always noticed . . .
Thank you.

LINDA DANO

To Trip, who definitely has style

ANNE KYLE

G. P. Putnam's Sons
Publishers Since 1838
200 Madison Avenue
New York, NY 10016

The author gratefully acknowledges permission to reprint
material from The Bonios Plan™ on pages 178–181.
© The Bonios Plan, Inc., 1995. All rights reserved.
Published by Chatham Institute, Inc., 127 Main Street,
Chatham, NJ 07928; (800) 760-5490.

Library of Congress Cataloging-in-Publication Data

Dano, Linda.
Looking great . . . : fashion authority and television star
Linda Dano shares her style and beauty secrets to help you
look your best / Linda Dano with Anne Kyle.
p.   cm.
ISBN 0-399-14272-X
I. Clothing and dress. 2. Fashion. 3. Beauty, Personal.
I. Kyle, Anne. II. Title.
TT507.D28   1997   96-39124 CIP
646.7'042—dc21
Printed in the United States of America
5   7   9   10   8   6   4

This book is printed on acid-free paper. ∞

Book design by Judith Stagnitto Abbate

Acknowledgments

I want to say thank you to all of you who have helped me arrive at where I am now. It's been a long, difficult journey, full of pain and joy and the love of so many.

To Anne Kyle, my partner and cowriter of this book: Thank you—you made the mental blocks disappear. To Denise Silvestro, my editor at Putnam: It's been fun when I thought it would be so hard. To Jimmy Vines, my agent: Agents aren't supposed to be so wonderful. To Jonathan Pillot, my advisor and friend: Thank you—it was your vision and you made it happen. To Vivien Stern: Thank you for everyday—you make it all so effortless. To my dear friends Barbara Sperling, Jill Farren Phelps, Jeanette Grewenig, who always encourage me and make me feel I can do anything. To Euclides Coutinho, who takes such good care of us—thank you, I have many less worries with you in my life. And to all of those who have affected me, taught me, advised me—and believed in me: my parents, my Grandmother Myrtle, my brother, Jack, my kids and grandkids and family, Nina Blanchard, Edie Locke, my friends on *Attitudes* and *Another World*, designers and artists whom I have had the pleasure of knowing. And last, to my husband and friend, Frank Attardi: Thank you for your support, advice, encouragement, and love—I can do all things with you next to me.

— LINDA DANO

A book doesn't get written by itself, and many people have contributed to the completion of this one. Their help has been invaluable and deserves my sincere thanks. From start to finish, they are: Jimmy Vines, Lisa Collier Cool, Jonathan Pillot, Vivien Stern, Shawne Cooper, Nina Blanchard, Bonnie Fuller, Anne Hardy, Dr. Thomas Romo, Dr. Steven J. Pearlman, Will Park, Rosie O'Donnell, Jackée, and Leeza Gibbons.

I am especially grateful for the hard work of our editor, Denise Silvestro, at Putnam. Her favorite phrase, "I'll take care of that for you," was always music to my ears.

And finally, thank you to my new friend Linda Dano, probably the nicest person in show business.

— ANNE KYLE

Contents

Part III. Beauty

Part IV. Self-Image

Introduction

Some say that style is like rhythm: you're either born with it or you're not. I don't believe that. You *can* learn to put clothes together, apply makeup, and create a lovely environment to live in. You just have to learn how. You call a plumber to fix a broken toilet because you don't know how to do it yourself. That doesn't mean you can't learn to fix a toilet; you're certainly smart enough, you just never wanted to learn. It's the same thing with style. If you want to learn the secrets, I'll tell you. And with a little practice, you can do it: you can stop making style mistakes, gain confidence, and improve every aspect of your life.

Of course, I have a little bit of an advantage because I learned at the knee of a master. My mother has always made looking and feeling good a top priority. Even now, I love shopping with her. Although at eighty-five she's slowed down a bit, it's still fun. But when I was growing up in Long Beach, California, we didn't have any money. Certainly not any extra money to spend on

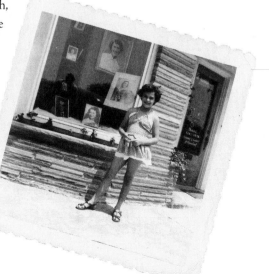

Me at age eight. I can't believe I ever wore anything this revealing!

clothes. Still, I was always the best-dressed girl in my class because my mother would weed through piles of fabric until she found just the piece she was looking for, bring it home, and sew it into a stylish outfit for me. Like the Christmas I needed a coat. Now, I knew we didn't have money for a new coat. I resigned myself to the fact that I probably wouldn't get one. But my mother saved enough to buy the fabric and *made* me one. It was a very difficult project, as anyone who sews knows, but she worked on it until she figured it out. It just goes to show you that when you really try, you can learn things that you never thought you could.

It also shows you that you don't need a gazillion dollars to pull together a fabulous wardrobe. I'm not suggesting that you need to take up sewing to get the look you want, but there are ways to keep down costs. I can afford to buy pretty much anything I want at this stage of my life, but I really don't buy much. Or I should say, too much. That's because when you have a closet, and drawers, and probably the closet in the guest bedroom, too, stuffed with clothes and shoes and accessories, you can never find anything to wear. You have so much stuff that's not organized you may not even know what you have and what you need. For example, let's say you have a great outfit that you need a brown belt for. But you can't find the brown belt, or maybe you never bought one. And every time you go shopping you forget to buy a brown belt. So you never wear this great outfit, all because you don't have the stupid belt. This is the stuff that takes practice: weeding out what you don't wear, what you'll never wear, and replacing it with something that you'll wear all the time (and having all the stuff that goes with it).

Makeup and hair and all the other things that go into looking great above the shoulders is something that confuses a lot of women. They're *afraid* of it. Have you ever seen a fifty-year-old woman who has the same hairstyle she had when she was twenty? It doesn't look so hot anymore, but she doesn't know how to update her look so she does nothing. Big mistake. Hair will grow back and makeup can be wiped off. It's worth it to experiment a little bit and take the chance that something new will work better. It may not even be a new cut that our Peggy Sue needs. She might try adding a hairpiece—they're terrific these

1953—*me and Mom (she made the clothes).*

Nina Blanchard (the agent) asked me to take some snapshots so she could see if I was photogenic—my mother gets photo credit on this one. This shot launched my modeling career— scary, huh?

days—for a night out, or maybe one of the new wash-out hair dyes. You may look fabulous as a redhead! There are lots of things you can do to alter your look without making drastic, or permanent, changes. I know about all of these tricks because I have seen them used for over thirty years by professional stylists. Why do you think that actresses always look so great on TV and in films? It's because they have a team of artists who know how to create individual styles just for them. You can do the same thing. You just have to find what works.

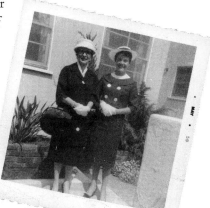

I have a simple solution that I use on bad hair days. One day I was having a really, really bad hair day, so I just threw on a beret and pulled it down on one side so that it slanted across my forehead. I looked in the mirror and went, "Aha, this actually looks like I intended to wear a beret today. It adds some style." I don't knit, but I found someone to make these little hats in every color for only a few dollars a piece. When I buy a new outfit, I order a beret to match. Everyone thinks I wear them because they look great and match my outfit, when really they are covering my limp hair. Even though I started wearing them to hide under, they've become a part of my personal style. I get extra points for having bad hair!

Me and Mom all dressed up—probably the beginning of my love affair with hats.

As an actress, I am well aware of the effects of aging. Looks are a big factor in my business. Fortunately, I seem to be aging well, but I have also always been very careful about my skin and not exposing it to bad elements. Now luckily there are wonderful products to protect and revitalize damaged skin. I have gotten this far on my beauty regimen alone, but I have to admit that I am not beyond going for plastic surgery. Some may be appalled by that, but I say, go for whatever is going to make you feel better about yourself. A little collagen injected in the right places can go a long way. Unfortunately, finding a good plastic surgeon takes some research. I've done it for you. I have discovered all of the little nips and tucks available to women, and also how to go about it safely. I know how to find a reputable surgeon, how much each procedure costs, and how much down time you'll have. All things you'll need to know before going under the knife.

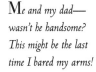

The big beauty issue for me has always been my weight. I am sure there is a 300-pound woman inside of me dying to get out. I love food. Love to buy it, make it, and mostly love to eat it. Yet I managed to lose thirty-five pounds and maintain a

Me and my dad—wasn't he handsome? This might be the last time I bared my arms!

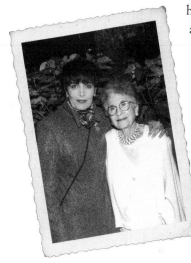

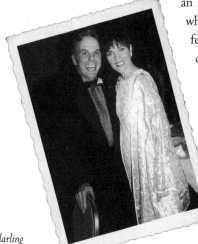

healthy weight. I used to think that if I was a very good girl—and I was—I could eat anything I wanted. Of course, eating made me feel bad, so it was a real catch-22. What I've learned is that I can have my cake, just make sure it's small, and don't eat the whole bloody thing! I can teach you how to stop depriving yourself and lose weight without using diet pills or liquid diets. It worked for me!

Okay, now that you're slender, perfectly dressed, made-up, and coiffed, why do you still feel crummy? A lot is expected of women these days. Not only are you supposed to make the bacon, bring it home and cook it, and serve it in a pretty cocktail dress, you still have to bathe the kids, get them in bed, make lunches for the next day, bring them to daycare, run to the gym and somehow find time to have sex with your husband. Whew! No wonder you're exhausted. In a sense, women really haven't come that far. You're still putting yourself last. And that's not fair. It's important to your—and your family's—well-being to take some time out for yourself. It's easier for me because I've never had kids of my own and I have Frank, who is an extremely supportive husband, but my schedule is probably just as hectic as yours. I've had to learn that the world won't fall apart if I take an afternoon (or even an hour) just for myself. And guess what? My world is actually better when I disappear for a few hours to browse through an antique shop or hide in a corner to read a book. Yours can be, too.

It's been a long and bumpy ride through thirty years of show business, but thank goodness I learned *something*. Come along and let me share it with you.

— L I N D A D A N O

Me and my mother—she still looks fabulous at eighty-five, doesn't she? And yes, I am very proud of her!

Me and my darling Frank—we really are as happy as we look! (Courtesy Gary M. Czvekus)

Part I

Getting Started

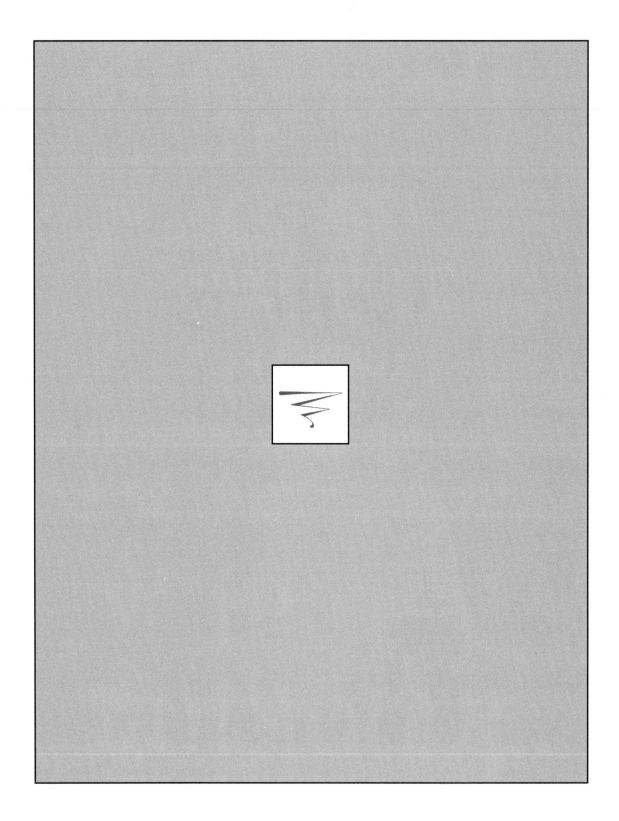

Chapter 1

You're the Picture . . . Frame It

I remember the exact moment when I realized that dressing well would make a huge difference in how people saw me, and eventually, how I saw myself. Did that ever happen to you? *My defining moment was my junior-high-school graduation dance.* As the big day approached and I had nothing to wear, my mother planned an information-gathering excursion to the best stores in Long Beach, California, where we lived when I was growing up. You see, we didn't have the money to just walk into a store and buy the perfect dress. My mother would have to make it. That meant waltzing into stores as if we owned them and scouting out the best styles. We would take dresses into the fitting room and my mother would investigate every seam until she memorized how the dress was put together.

Well, we finally saw *the* dress in the window of an expensive boutique. By the time we got to the dressing room, I was shaking from fear. I knew that any minute we would be found out and embarrassed (and there was no doughnut store nearby to comfort me). *The* dress was a little black number with a sheer top. It looked absolutely divine on me. And for me to say that . . . oh, boy! All of a sudden, I was another person. No matter what the truth was, my whole life I had always believed I looked fat. Unbelievably, in this dress I looked thin and like the person who could afford such an expensive outfit. My mother went through the usual routine of examining every stitch on the dress and writing down measurements. And then, with our faces red and our hearts pounding, we lied and told the saleswoman that it didn't fit, and practically ran out of the store.

We found the fabric—I was so thrilled—and my mother went home and made an exact copy of the dress. When I walked into the graduation dance my friends looked at me as if I were a different person. Honest to God, a different person. The way they responded to me made a lasting impression. It was the dress that gave me the confidence. They were seeing a girl with style and confidence; one that existed only in *the* dress. I can still conjure up that feeling. It has affected me to this day. I knew that I was still the same insecure Linda Rae Wildermuth inside, but in *the* dress I felt different. I felt special. I felt pretty. I wanted to feel that way forever. Right then I decided I would always find the money to dress well, somehow. I would work on myself from the outside in. I would create a frame for the picture of me. I used clothes to make me feel great even when I didn't. Once I had the confidence in knowing I looked great, I could devote more time to developing my personality and talents. Over the years, I have slowly filled in the pieces of my picture so that the me you see on the outside—confident, stylish, smart—is closer to who I really am.

So what does that mean? It means that the clothes *can* make the woman. They can make you. But first you have to find out who you are and analyze why you dress the way you do. What do you like about the way you dress? What do you like about the way other people dress? What don't you like? Once we uncover the layers of your fashion psyche, the hard part is done. So . . . let's get down to work.

What Type Are You?

Most women base their wardrobe on their body and how they feel about it. Do you think you're fat (who doesn't?) and wear clothes that are way too big? Guess what? That just makes you look even bigger! Do you hate your thighs, or breasts, or some other part, and dress to cover, cover, cover? Do you lack confidence and choose plain styles that do *nothing* for you? Worst of all, are you still trying to please your mother, your husband, or, God forbid, trying to look like the most popular girl in tenth grade? You can probably find yourself somewhere in the above list, but let's define you even more. We'll do it by playing a game. Read the descriptions below and choose the one or two (or—horrors!—all) fashion types that fit the way—and reasons—you dress. This is like anything else: Once you identify the problem it is really easy to fix. I promise, it won't hurt a bit.

Little Girl Syndrome

WHAT YOU DO: You wear the clothes that other people like, and probably even buy for you. You dressed for your mother and then for your husband, but have never evolved into finding *your* style. Mom loved those Peter Pan collars so you wore them well into adulthood. Your husband prefers tight skirts and high heels. You want to please him, so even though you hate those clothes (and boy, are they uncomfortable) you wear them anyway.

WHAT IT MEANS: You have not come into your own yet. You're not acknowledging who *you* are and not letting your style reflect your sense of self. It's always about pleasing someone else, not you. It's easier to not put up a fight, isn't it? But what you're saying through your clothes is that you don't think you're anybody. That your ideas don't count.

WHAT YOU NEED TO DO: The hardest part about changing this syndrome is that the people you have worked so hard to please may not like it. After all, they'll have to let go of the control they have over you. But you have to say to yourself, over and over again, that your clothes should show who *you* are, not who anyone else thinks you are or ought to be. You can create the frame for your picture, just like I did, by slowly integrating your fashion choices into your wardrobe. Really, no one is going to leave you just because you are wearing a perfectly tailored pantsuit instead of a poufy blouse and jumper. But when you start allowing your style to reflect the true you, the first thing you'll notice is that your personality will begin to come out of hiding. Hey, they may not like it, but then again, they may love the new you even more.

It may take a while to know who you even are, so first you should go with your instincts. Do you really like it? It it comfortable? Do you feel pretty? You'll make mistakes. That's okay. You're testing the waters and it takes time to say hello to the real you.

Seeing the Light

Soap-opera and sitcom star Judith Light was a client of my wardrobe-consulting business. Now, you know her as a beautiful, talented actress who always looks terrific. But in her private life she was a classic victim of Little Girl Syndrome. Her mother always bought her cute little ruffly blouses and dresses with cap sleeves (poufed cap sleeves!). After she was on her own and buying her own clothes, she continued to mimic her mother's sense of style. As a result, she was a gorgeous adult dressing like a very cute ten-year-old girl.

You don't know how difficult it was to get her to part with these clothes. She would say, "Well, I'll just save this blouse to wear when I'm painting." I said, "Forget it." I knew she would have that blouse on as soon as I walked out the door. My job was to try to create a new look for her that would express her personality, not her mother's. The blouse went.

Of course, now Judith dresses beautifully. Not only does she look great all of the time, she feels great, too. That's because her clothes frame her personality perfectly. ✳

Shopaholic

WHAT YOU DO: You buy. Boy, do you buy. It doesn't matter if you can ever wear it, you buy it anyway. You may not even have a place to put it once you get it home, but you buy it anyway. Then you go to get dressed and you have nothing to wear. Except maybe shoes. Shopaholics always seem to have gorgeous shoes. I guess if you've bought every pair ever made, it's not so hard to find a pair to wear. You may shop so much that your credit cards are maxed out and you're in deep debt.

WHAT IT MEANS: For you, the thrill is the act of shopping, not the building of a wardrobe. You may be lacking in other areas of your life and shopping fulfills a need. Shopping because you have to means you are out of control, comparable in the worst cases to an eating disorder. You just don't know who you are and think that maybe the item you buy today will change your life. Trust me, it won't.

WHAT YOU NEED TO DO: Mild cases can be cured by hiring a personal shopper or wardrobe consultant (our goal here is to build a wardrobe, right?) to weed through the mess in your closet and see if there is anything in there that you can actually wear. Without even looking in your closet, I would bet almost everything that there are lots of things that you can keep and build on. We need to start with the basics, and most of us already have them; we just don't recognize them.

I like to make lists. Now, be prepared, this is a lot of work. Go through your closet and put things in categories (see Chapter 2: Paring Down for details): First put shirts together, skirts together, and so on. Then get more detailed and move clothes into color groupings. Don't forget to separate day from evening, summer from winter. Decide what you will need to buy to make complete outfits. Write them down. This will take a while, but once you've done that, you get to the fun part: You get to go shopping to build on the clothes you already own. But now you'll go

Simple Works Best

Lots of women feel they have weight problems—and many do. A typical overweight woman will either never shop or shop *a lot*. If that's you, you're either in denial or in constant search for that one outfit that will change the way you look. What generally happens is that you then have a closet full of clothes that almost work, but not entirely.

My friend Rosie O'Donnell, the comedienne and talk-show host, has always been a little chubby and used to do the same things you do. Now that she's a mom and hosts a daily TV talk show, she doesn't have the time to devote to her clothes, so she got smart. "I have this guy who made me about ten suits that look great on me. They're all dark colors, which are best on me. I just grab a blouse and one of these suits and I know that I look the best I can."

Now you may think, *Hey, she's a star, she can afford to have her clothes custom-made.* But I'll bet she spent less on those ten suits than you do buying clothes off the rack that you never wear. Rosie really gets her money's worth because she wears her clothes. ✳

shopping with goals in mind. Buy only what's on the list. If you can't control yourself, make sure your personal shopper is with you and approves your purchases.

If you are in serious debt and can't control your spending, you need to get real help. See a therapist, call Debtors Anonymous, cut up credit cards. Do it now, today, right this minute. Buying just to buy is not going to improve your life—or how you look—it's just going to put you in debt and in trouble.

Sale Addict

WHAT YOU DO: We are *all* guilty of this: You scout the sale racks and get the very best deals. Problem is, you're buying junk. So what if it's puce and a little snug? It was on sale! As a matter of fact you have a closet full of great bargains—some still with tags attached—that are unwearable for one reason or another.

WHAT IT MEANS: It means you have no idea what you are doing. You're making buying decisions based on price alone. That's never a good idea because style goes right out the window. You don't have enough confidence to spend more money on the one thing that might look great on you. You think, *If I spend a lot and then I don't like it, I'm going to feel really bad. But if it's on sale, I'll just feel a little bad.*

WHAT YOU NEED TO DO: If you can't make full-price purchases because you're afraid of failure, get some help. Personal shoppers in department stores are free, and if you don't call them for help, they'll just sit in their offices all day doing nothing. You'll be doing them a favor. In my experience the women (and they are almost all women) who perform this service are always nice and friendly. They really do want to help and are good at what they do. They know the store and its merchandise and can quickly figure out who you are. Don't be intimidated by them. You don't have to spend thousands of dollars. Their job is to help you, *for free.*

It's a Steal

I once took a friend to a Donna Karan showroom sale. That's when you can go right to the workroom of the designer and buy leftover stock for amazing prices. My friend came running up to show me a huge men's jacket that she thought she had to have. It wasn't a flattering style and didn't even button properly, but still, she said, "Can you believe the price? And it's Donna Karan!"

Well, I *could* believe the price. Obviously this jacket wasn't a big seller in the stores, otherwise it wouldn't be here in the first place. There is a reason that things go on sale. One time in a million you can find the perfect bargain, but mostly things are on sale because no one liked them enough to buy them. If no one else liked them, you shouldn't get stuck with them either.

Needless to say, I talked my friend out of buying the jacket that would have hung in the back of her closet until she threw it out, I'm sure still crying, "But it's Donna Karan!" ✳

It's still okay to weed through the sale racks, but you can't buy anything unless it's the right color, style, and it fits. And as a side note, it must be something you need. What is missing from your wardrobe? Is that great sale item on your list? You have to say, "I'm missing a black shirt and if I don't find it, I am *not* going to buy something else. I will just go to the next store until I find the black shirt." Those are the rules.

Age-Impaired

WHAT YOU DO: You're a grown woman now—with grown-up responsibilities—and yet you still hang on to your micro-minis and crop tops. Some days you wear fishnet hose with satin shorts. You wear a little too much makeup, your neckline is a little too low and your belt a little too wide for your age-affected thickening waist. You want desperately to be fifteen years younger than you are, but you're hurt and surprised when others don't take you seriously.

WHAT IT MEANS: Mostly it means you look silly. I'll take it a step further. I think it looks sad. Dressing like a teenager screams out that you don't know who you are, and that you don't have enough self-esteem to dress your age. You don't like where you are. You don't like your life right now. Dressing this way also means that you want people to notice you. They will notice you—boy, will they notice you—but not for any of the right reasons.

What's happened is that somewhere through the years you stopped. You stopped at a particular year you liked. Probably when great things happened. You had a career, you got married, you had your kids. Maybe you were afraid to go forward because you'd lose all you had. You'd lose your youth. *It's all over,* you thought. Well, now it's time to move on.

There's that tired old adage that you must dress your age. Not necessarily true, but you should let your clothes say who you are today. Not yesterday and certainly not ten years from now.

WHAT YOU NEED TO DO: First, think about what you want to accomplish. Think about several things. *Who am I? What do I want to say about me? What do I want people to see when they first meet me? How do I want to be treated?* I know that you don't want to be treated with no regard, like a piece of fluff. I know that.

You can still wear young-looking clothes, just change the proportions. I don't like short-short skirts on most people, whether they're ten or one hundred, so first I'd say wear longer skirts. Wear solid-color hose instead of patterns. And, if in your heart and soul you still want to feel like a sexpot, save the skin-tight stuff for your husband in the bedroom. It'll be your secret to share.

Repeat Offender

WHAT YOU DO: Here's what you come home with from every shopping trip: a black jacket. If it's been a long day of shopping, you might have a black skirt and black pumps, too. You go to hang them up, and (wonders!) you find you already have ten black jackets and five skirts that are for the most part exactly the same as the one you just bought. When you dress you put on . . . hmmm . . . let me guess . . . a black skirt and jacket?

WHAT IT MEANS: You have no real identity. You are either so insecure about your fashion savvy that you continue to buy and wear the same thing, or you just don't care and figure you are safe wearing what you always wear (even if it's a new version of the same old thing). Your personality is not being expressed. You have no sense of adventure and individual style. I believe that you don't want anyone to notice you, so you play it really safe.

WHAT YOU NEED TO DO: First, choose one or two black outfits and donate the rest to charity. There must be a homeless model out there who needs some more black in her shopping cart. Second, put on one of your standard outfits and go shopping (call a personal shopper if you're unsure). Look for items that go with but don't duplicate what you already have. Because you have all the black you need, you're ahead of the game: Those are your basics! Add some color, a plaid or a print, go longer or shorter, try a different cut. Buy some accessories that have color.

After you bring your purchases home, you have to wear them. You might dress to go out and put on your new red jacket, take it off—STOP! Put it back on! Go! This is hard, almost like weaning a baby from a bot-

Adios, Mistakes!

Recently, I was in Puerto Rico with Frank, and we stopped in a small shoe store where I spotted the cutest strappy sandals. I picked them up and discovered that they were only $20 a pair! I sat down and tried them on, but then I didn't follow my own rules. I didn't walk around in them or even think about what they might go with. They were just so cute!

They were available in five colors, of which I bought four. Wow! Four pairs of shoes for eighty bucks! Do you know they are the most uncomfortable shoes I've ever had? I can hardly walk across the room. It would be fine if Frank could carry me everywhere, but even I am not that lucky.

They were a mistake and if I were smart, I would have thrown them out long ago because every time I look at them, I realize how stupid I was. You know what? . . . Give me a minute. . . . I am going right now to toss them out. There, I can't believe how much better I feel. ✳

tle. You have to tear yourself away from the familiar. You'll see, you'll love the re-sponse you'll get. So go ahead, take some chances. After all, they're only clothes.

Sweatshopper

WHAT YOU DO: You pull on any old thing. You wear leggings and big sweaters. You steal your husband's sweatpants and college T-shirt. This isn't about being comfy. This is about not caring. You feel crummy about the way you look, and do everything you can to hide. The clothes you wear feel comfortable, but they don't make you feel good about yourself.

WHAT IT MEANS: You put yourself last. You work to make sure that everyone else is taken care of, and you really don't have time to devote to building a wardrobe. You have low self-esteem and figure why bother, right? Wrong. You are important. Just ask all those people you take care of. I'll bet they would say that they really value what you do for them.

You may be denying you have a weight problem (but sweatshoppers can also be thin) or thinking in the back of your head that you'll start to care how you look when you've lost some weight. Why wait? Looking better will inspire you to lose weight faster. Invest in yourself now.

WHAT YOU NEED TO DO: Start loving yourself. If you can't do that, try lik-ing. You *are* allowed to feel good about yourself. If you don't, how can you expect anyone else to pay attention to you? I know . . . you say you don't want any attention, but I don't believe that. We all want—and need—to feel loved. Start slowly. Improve the way you dress just one day a week. Dress for yourself. Pick outfits that make you feel attractive. A great way to jump-start this makeover is to start wearing a little makeup, even if you're all alone. Go, right now, and put on a bit of mascara and some lipstick. You may do a double take every time you pass the mirror. *Who is that?* you'll think. That's a woman who cares about herself. A happier woman.

Many of the feelings associated with dressing in sweats and big sweaters have to do with weight. I know you don't love those extra pounds. And I know how hard it is to lose them too. But as you make each small change, you will gain the confidence to make the big ones. It's not easy, but look at you. You bought this book. You want to try, right? It can be done. Believe it.

Closet-Paralyzed

WHAT YOU DO: You're a little bit Shopaholic, a little bit Repeat Offender. You love to shop and have money to spend. You have closets full of beautiful clothes (many of them duplicates), but can never find *anything* to wear. So, of course, you must you go shopping again and buy more of what you'll never put on. You open your closet to look at all of your clothes and can't for the life of you figure out how to put them together.

WHAT IT MEANS: You're frustrated. You know you have the money to buy nice clothes, but can't seem to pull it off. *Why can't I look like so-and-so?* you think. I would guess that you are not good at making decisions in other parts of your life, either. I'm only guessing. I would also guess that you are not very organized. Are you that way in other areas of your life? Probably. It shouldn't come as a shock to you that you can never find anything to wear, because you're just buying clothes not building a wardrobe.

WHAT YOU NEED TO DO: You're like Marsha Mason in *The Goodbye Girl*. She picks a picture from a decorating magazine and tries to duplicate that look in her own living room. It's not really her style, and she doesn't have the expertise to pull it off. She keeps saying, "Elliot, what's wrong with this room? Why doesn't it look like the picture?" That's you. You're trying so hard to look like somebody else that you never look like you.

So here's the plan: Eliminate, eliminate, eliminate. I would bring a friend or a wardrobe consultant into your closet. It can be anyone who has the strength to get you to pare down. (Go back to SALE ADDICT, make lists, organize your closet, learn what you have and what you need.) I know you will uncover some real treasures that are worth saving and building on. But first get rid of the mistakes. Don't beat yourself up; we all make mistakes. If we're smart, we put them behind us and move on. If you have the money to buy all

She Had to Have It

I once had a client of my wardrobe-consulting business who was totally Closet-Paralyzed. Her shopping style was more about acquiring things than building a wardrobe. Of course, her closets were stuffed to the gills, yet she never really looked her best because she didn't know how to coordinate her clothing.

I was checking out the new trends in New York's Bergdorf Goodman's one day when I bumped into her. I was dressed in a complete ensemble, right down to a custom-made knit hat. My client ran up to me and asked to buy the entire outfit, top to bottom, jewelry included, right off my back. Right then. She didn't care if I went home naked, she had to have the whole thing. She begged! I knew it was just a passing hysteria, but it made her crazy that she couldn't have this outfit. I said no and tried to urge her to buy clothes that would look good on *her*, but I never totally cured her of her compulsive shopping. ✳

of these clothes, surely you can afford a professional to help you sort out and build a new wardrobe. One that you'll actually enjoy wearing, not one that wears you.

Size-Deluded

WHAT YOU DO: Those afflicted with this problem are usually overweight (or think they are). You buy big, baggy clothes because you think they will hide those extra pounds. The clothes are slightly better than the Sweatshopper would buy, but not much. You are hiding underneath a tent and hoping no one will notice. But they will notice. They'll notice that you are sloppy and don't care about the way you look. So not only will you still look overweight, you'll look disheveled, too. The flip side of this is buying clothes a size too small, thinking that you'll lose weight. How many of us have done that? You never lose the weight, though, and you wear the clothes anyway. They're uncomfortable and you are, too.

WHAT IT MEANS: By hiding under tents or squeezing into too small clothes, you are not acknowledging that you have a weight problem. This is a tough one. I know. When I am heavy, I don't care how I look, at first. I just think, *Oh well, I'm fat again, I might as well look as bad as I feel.* That happens to you, too, right? Some days you just hate yourself and can't get over it. If you feel this way, you're probably trying to hide and hope you can just get through the day without eating ten doughnuts.

WHAT YOU NEED TO DO: Buy the right size. I have never understood why bigger women feel that they don't have a right to buy nice clothes that fit them well. This is your figure. Hiding it won't change it. Stop punishing yourself for being overweight and go shopping. Many designers have finally started to recognize that large-size women deserve flattering fashions. You will be surprised to see the improved selections. If you're dressing-room shy, then catalog shop (see CATALOG SHOPPING, page 59) or buy clothes that can be tried on at home and returned.

If you plan to lose weight, do it *before* buying a whole new wardrobe. It never works the other way around. By the time you've lost weight, the clothes you've bought may be out of style or season. They may not even look good on the new you. Save your shopping treat until you are a size you know you can maintain. But that doesn't mean you should wait until you're thin to wear nice clothes. Do it today, but wear nice clothes that fit you *now.*

Color-Blind

WHAT YOU DO: This is another area where larger women err. You wear big prints and loud colors. You even mix them. You're trying to dazzle, but you really only make people dizzy. You probably also wear shiny fabrics, which make you look like a headlight. You're timing might be off, too. Do you wear velvets and brocades during the day? Glitz to the office? Probably.

WHAT IT MEANS: You are crying out for attention. *Look at me, look at me! Take that,* you say. *I can wear what ever I want.* You can, but that doesn't mean you look good. You think that because you're large you'll never look chic so you might as well grab attention any way possible.

WHAT YOU NEED TO DO: It's pretty obvious, isn't it? You're getting the attention you crave, but it's not because people think you look great; it's because they're blinded by your bright lights. Your clothes shouldn't be brighter than your personality. In my opinion, large women *can't* wear everything (most people can't wear *every*thing). You need to tone it down and find styles that are flattering for you. Dig deep and find the confidence to show the world who you really are by thinking more about your fashion choices. People are more likely to overlook your weight and respond positively when you wear a more pulled-together, quieter look. I have friends who are large ladies, and they represent that big truly can be beautiful. Remember, often a whisper is heard more clearly than a shout.

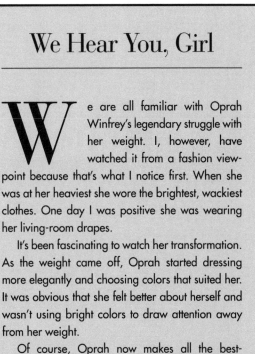

We Hear You, Girl

We are all familiar with Oprah Winfrey's legendary struggle with her weight. I, however, have watched it from a fashion viewpoint because that's what I notice first. When she was at her heaviest she wore the brightest, wackiest clothes. One day I was positive she was wearing her living-room drapes.

It's been fascinating to watch her transformation. As the weight came off, Oprah started dressing more elegantly and choosing colors that suited her. It was obvious that she felt better about herself and wasn't using bright colors to draw attention away from her weight.

Of course, Oprah now makes all the best-dressed lists; but she spent years on the other side, enduring snide jokes about her appearance. You can learn a lesson from her. ✹

What Now?

You've read the previous pages and have discovered that you are a walking fashion disaster. You see yourself, at least a little bit, in all of the fashion personalities. I've made you crazy, and you now have even less of an idea of how you should dress. Don't hate me! This is a process, and I'll see you through until the end. At least now you know what can go wrong, even with the best intentions. Don't worry, there is a method to my madness. I believe—no, I *know*—dressing well requires a plan and then some work. You've taken the first step by buying this book. By the time we're done, you'll have confidence to spare.

Chapter 2

Paring Down

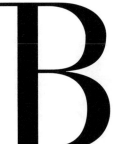efore you can even begin building and
maintaining a solid wardrobe, you will need to go through all
of your closets and drawers to get rid of everything you don't
or can't wear. Here we will work on organizing your closet so
that, at a glance, you can see its contents and pull together an
outfit in seconds. When we're done, you'll know what you
have, what you need, and where everything is.

  This is an important step, which might take you hours to
complete, so set aside a chunk of time when you know you won't be disturbed, and
you'll be able to finish the job. You don't want to leave this project half done. It's better to have a disorganized closet than to have all of your belongings strewn around
your bedroom for a few weeks until you find time to reorganize. You'll just lose all
incentive. So dig in, and I promise by the time we're finished, you will not only be
cured of being Closet-Paralyzed, you will know exactly what you need to complete
your wardrobe. (This is where I totally believe in rewards. Promise yourself something great when you finish this job. Eat a hot fudge sundae. With no guilt.)

  I can't tell you how many times I have stumbled upon a great lost outfit which
I've missed out on wearing because I forgot I had it. Does that sound familiar? *Oh,
there's that brown wool suit!* Of course, by the time I've spotted it, it's summer and a

brown wool suit is about as useful as a parka. I try very hard now to keep a close eye on my closets and do a thorough reorganization every season. I even do a little tweaking throughout a season. It can get away from me if I don't. Just like anything else, the first time you do this it will take awhile, but if you keep it up, you'll see that it gets easier and easier.

Lost in Space

You open the door to your closet and . . . wow! . . . it *really* is a mess. Hanging in one spot are the five outfits that you wear every week. Next are some blouses, a few skirts, more blouses . . . and look . . . back there . . . a dress you've had since high school. What's that doing there? You never wear it (at least, I hope you don't); as a matter of fact, your eye tends to skip right over it. It's just always been there. You think, *I've saved it this long, I can't possibly throw it out now.* I've got news for you . . . it's going. If you are really going to do this, and I know you are, you have to realize that sentiment is not a good enough reason to pack your closet full of useless items. (If you absolutely must save a special outfit, pack it away in a box. Just get it out of your closet).

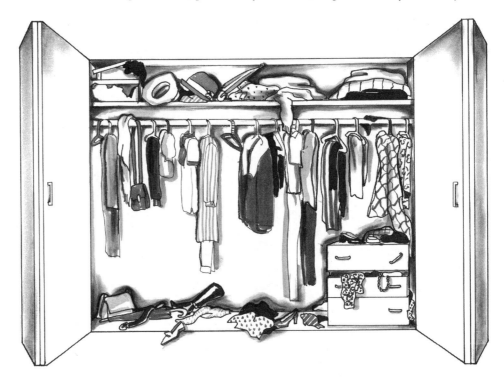

For inspiration, decide ahead of time where you are going to donate all of your old clothes. Choose a women's shelter, Goodwill, or even a little sister. As you toss each item into the reject bag think about how much use a less fortunate person will get from your castoffs. You'll benefit, too. When you donate, obtain a receipt (the amount is the market value of the clothes—it adds up) and make sure you deduct the amount from your income tax.

Now, let's get to work. Go through each item in your closet and check it for fit and damage. If something is too big, decide if it is worth tailoring to fit. Will you wear it then? If not, toss it. If something is too small, really think: Are you going to lose weight or do you just hope to? Keep clothes that fit you now. If you just can't bear to get rid of all of your skinny clothes, hang them in another closet or pack them away in a box. As you get better at paring down, you will also become more realistic about what you can actually wear. You'll probably save things during this round that will be edited out next time.

Make one pile for items you want to keep but that need repairs. Are buttons missing? Does a zipper stick? Are seams separating? Of course, you will have to make the repairs or take things to a tailor. No fair just making a pile and leaving it there. Add to this group skirts that need a hemline adjustment and anything that is too large but that you want to keep. If you can't make the repairs yourself and don't know a good tailor, check with your local dry cleaner. They usually have a person that performs this service and may not charge as much as a tailor, who depends on sewing for all of her income. A typical fee for a hem is about $10 to $15. Reattaching buttons, replacing zippers, and fixing tears cost only a few dollars. Tailoring a too-large jacket will cost more because of the work involved, so make sure you love that jacket or can't replace it more cheaply.

Start with Things That Hang

Every article of clothing now hanging in your closet is in good condition and fits, so all you have to do is go through the rest until you are left with items that you like and that you'll wear. Getting rid of clothes is hard. After all, you paid good money for them. Some are still like new. Remember the big tax deduction you'll be getting and then follow these rules:

✹   If you don't trust your own opinion, get a friend to help. Open a bottle of wine, put on some upbeat music, and make it a party. Offer to do the same for her.

✳ Don't ask your boyfriend/husband to be that friend unless he has an undisputed sense of style. Otherwise, the man in your life will not have a clue as to how you should shape your wardrobe. ("But, honey, you look great in those pink hotpants . . .")

✳ Follow the twelve-month rule: If you haven't worn it for a year, out it goes. It doesn't matter if you love it, paid a lot for it, or you just know you'll wear it someday . . . toss it.

✳ This should go without saying, but I'll say it anyway: Get rid of anything that still has the price tag attached.

✳ Edit similar items. Do you really need five black jackets? If they really are different and you wear each one to complete an outfit, by all means, keep every one. But if they are all lightweight tuxedo jackets, keep two. Okay, three (but review again next season to see if you can get by with two).

✳ Have you outgrown certain styles? I don't mean by weight, I mean by age. Is it time to get rid of your minis? Do you really feel comfortable wearing a formfitting dress? If you're hanging on to stuff because you don't want to grow up, then you have to, well, grow up. You'll look just as good (better) in age-appropriate clothes . . . I promise.

Even the Pros Do It

———

You may wonder how soap-opera wardrobe departments organize and store all of the clothes that the dozens of cast members wear. They do it just like you and I. A few times a year, they go through everything and weed out clothes that they know we won't wear again. Anything too damaged to fix or out-of-date is removed and collected for an in-house sale. Special outfits—such as distinctive evening gowns—are also taken out of circulation because viewers will notice and say, "She's wearing *that* again!" Of course, the costumers keep many more clothes than we would have in our own closets, but they are all organized by color and season and character. The same rules apply, just on a larger scale. ✳

Shoes, Accessories, and Other Space Hogs

Shoes hold a special place in every woman's heart. We all have way too many, myself included. Men don't get it. When Imelda Marcos was on trial, all the press could talk about were her 5,000 pairs of shoes. Men thought, *Gee, she could have bought a Corvette with all that money.* I, and most women, thought, *What a lucky duck.* Shoes are a "feel good" sort of purchase that we can understand. When we're feeling fat, bloated, or just can't find anything else to buy, the shoe department is where we head. You don't need to lose ten pounds to fit into a pair. We can buy shoes right now. And we do. Problem is, they take up a lot of space. And if we're honest, we know that we really only wear a few favorite pairs. Paring down shoes is very hard. If you have the space, by all means keep them all. If not, go through the same steps listed above.

Nothing looks worse than damaged or torn shoes. So even if they're your very favorite pair, they may have to go. (Do check in stores—or with the manufacturer— to see if you can replace them.) Take damaged shoes to a shoemaker and ask if they can be made to look like new. A replacement sole will run about $20 per pair. For just a heel or toe, expect to pay about $10. Torn seams are the easiest to repair and may cost only a few dollars. Sometimes all that is needed is a good cleaning and shine, which you can do yourself. This is worth doing, because you are more apt to wear shoes that look shiny and new. You'll expand your repertoire and save money.

Check the fit on shoes, too. "Ah, now I remember why I never wear these shoes," you'll say as you squeeze your toes into a too-narrow style. Also, even though you may think your shoe size doesn't change, it does. If you've recently gained weight or had a baby, your foot could have grown a full size.

Scarves, belts, and hats have a way of making their way to the back of your closet and disappearing. You'll probably find some treasures back there after you've removed all of your clothes. Again, check for damage. And here's some good news . . . finally! Since these items take up little space—when stored properly—you can probably keep most of them. Accessories are what personalize your look; they make your outfits unique, and they add a lot of versatility to your wardrobe. At the end of this chapter, after we go through your drawers and other secret hiding places, I'll tell you how to rebuild your closet so that you have room for everything.

Do Shoes Grow?

After I lost thirty-five pounds I discovered that I also lost inches everywhere, including my feet. I would never have believed this if I didn't see it myself. My feet were a solid size ten and now they're a 9½. I have packed away all of my tens at home, but Felicia is still walking around on the set looking like Minnie Mouse. Check out my feet when you're watching *Another World*. Felicia clops around between the bookstore and the hospital because the wardrobe department still believes she's a size ten. ✴

Sweaters, Socks, Underwear, and Everything Else You Have Crammed into Your Dresser

Drawers are great for hiding things . . . and messes. You just push down as hard as you can and push the drawer closed. Nobody has to know what's in there. Including you. Cleaning out your dresser may take you a while, so you'll be tempted to tackle it another day, but don't. You'll need to see what's in there to check if hose match suits or if you have the strapless bra needed for an evening dress. In TV costume departments the dressers always hang complete outfits together. You should, too, because it makes it easier to pull together an outfit—and it's more likely that you'll wear it if all the extras are right there.

There's no pretty way to do this, so just dump out drawers one at a time. Again, follow the rules above and check for damaged items. Some things to remember:

* Check sweaters for pulls or moth holes. Put damaged items in repair pile. Some tailors are experts at matching thread and weave, so don't assume a wool sweater is a goner until you've asked around.

* Check T-shirts and turtlenecks for tears and stains. Light-colored cottons tend to yellow over time, so put aside a pile to be bleached. Decide on their fate after they've been brightened. NOTE: Even expensive cottons can be bleached. Too much dry-cleaning can leave whites gray, so I bleach them at home every once in a while and then take them to the cleaners for a good pressing. Bleach in the hottest water you have for best results.

Neatness Counts

Ages ago, I shared a dressing room on *Another World* with television star Jackée. I've always loved the way she defines herself—she has her own style. I asked her to tell us all how she does it. It's funny, I am finding that the best-dressed women keep it so simple.

Jackée buys whole outfits when she shops and keeps them hung together in her closet. She says she has tons of clothes, but that's okay because they're organized. Her closet is arranged by color and type of clothing (dresses in one place, jackets and slacks in another, etc.) so she can dash in and select an outfit in a flash.

Her many, many pairs of shoes are stored in their boxes. "I take a Polaroid picture of them as soon as I bring them home and tape it to the side of the box. That way shoes stay neat and I can instantly see what's in each box without making a mess."

Knowing where your clothes are is half the battle in putting them together and achieving the style you know you have. *

✽ Pitch all single socks. I know it breaks your heart. Mine, too. (I swear that my dog Charlie is eating one sock at a time just to drive me crazy.) You don't really believe that the dryer is going to someday cough up the match, do you? Somehow I do. But I pitch singles anyway.

✽ Slide a hand into pantyhose and stockings to check for runs. Toss pairs with obvious runs. Some people will advise you to salvage torn pantyhose by cutting off the damaged leg of two pairs and wearing them together. I could never really master this because I can't remember which pairs are cut up and I end up spending fifteen minutes rooting through my drawer. In my opinion, it's better to splurge a little in this area and always wear close-to-perfect hose. Save in other places, and please, don't glob nail polish on your knee to stop a run. Buy a new pair.

✽ You truly only need seven pairs of regular underpants and seven standard bras. You can add a few pair of panties for when you have your period and specialized bras that go with certain outfits. Other than that, sorry, but out the rest go.

✽ Only you can decide what stays in your lingerie drawer. What's sexy to you is sexy to you. However, anything that is in bad shape or doesn't fit has to go.

Making It Right

Okay, so that's it, you've done it. You've worked hard and weeded out your wardrobe. Ready for a hot bath and that sundae? Not so fast. We have to organize and put everything back first. I believe that in order to dress well your closet has to be a nice place to visit. You can't be afraid to open the door. Everything has to be in its place and stored

Oops!

Even though I clean out my own closets every season, I still make mistakes all the time. When I married Frank in 1983, a lot of my life was in turmoil. It was the happiest time and the saddest. My only brother, Jack, was very ill with cancer, and neither he nor my parents could attend my wedding. Frank and I had set a Christmastime wedding date, so I thought I'd pull myself out of my funk by buying a cheery, red taffeta dress (this was my third wedding, after all!), which, looking back, was hideous on me. I look at the pictures and think, *Where is Linda, and what have you done with her?* At the time, I know I was thinking, *It's a Christmas wedding, this will be okay.* I thought the red dress would make me feel better, so I bought it, and wore it.

There is no excuse for what happened next. I continued to wear this awful dress to other functions. I just couldn't admit that I had made such a mistake. With my wedding dress no less! Every time I wore the dress and looked in the mirror, I thought, *You look awful in this dress, why don't you get rid of it?* I felt so stupid. Finally I came to my senses, had it dry-cleaned and now store it in my extra storage closet where I can see and touch it every now and then. What I'll never do again is *wear* it, so there's no point in having it take up space in my closet. ✽

in such a way that you can see it all. To make it that way you might need to call in a closet contractor or buy the poles, shelves, and special hooks to do it yourself. This expense is well worth it.

Having the right hangers for each one of your garments is important. They don't have to be expensive, but they do have to be the right shape. Clothes should be buttoned and zippered to maintain shape and prevent tears.

DRESSES

Hang dresses on plastic or wooden hangers that have rounded edges. Place them in the part of your closet where you have the most room underneath. If the bottom of your clothes is bunched up on top of shelves or shoe racks, they will wrinkle. I like to use padded hangers for such fine fabrics as silk because even the slightest edge leaves a bump in the shoulder.

SHIRTS AND BLOUSES

Casual or knit shirts (that don't wrinkle) should be folded and placed on a shelf or in a drawer. If the drawer is deep it makes sense to "file" them so you can see what you have. By file, I mean turn the stack on its side and place it in the drawer with the side edge facing up. You can also roll shirts and place them in drawers rolled end up. Arrange them in color order.

Hang blouses and shirts that wrinkle on curved plastic or wood hangers. Again, use padded hangers for delicates and arrange by color.

SKIRTS

You can either hang skirts singly on skirt hangers with clips—always look for rubber-coated clips—or buy a multitiered hanger and hang skirts together. If you have the space, I'd prefer to see them hanging one-by-one; often you lose sight of what's on a multitiered hanger because some skirts will be hidden from view. Exception: Keep suit skirts with jackets, hung underneath a two-part hanger with clips.

Finding Treasures

One of the greatest pleasures about cleaning out your closet will be discovering that you really do have some great clothes in there. I helped *Another World*'s executive producer, Jill Phelps, clean out her closet recently, and I was shocked to see what good taste she has. You see, I only see her in the two outfits she wears all the time. All along she's been buying—and shoving in her closet—stylish, wonderful clothes. She never wore them because she could never find them. She'd unpack her bags after a shopping trip and that would be the last she ever saw of those things. After we weeded out and reorganized, she discovered that she really didn't need to buy much to put together a terrific wardrobe. ✳

Jackets should always be hung on heavy wooden hangers that can support their weight. If they sag they will soon lose their shape. Separate by color and by season if you are going to keep year-round clothes in one closet. Leave pockets sewn shut to hold shape.

PANTS

Pants should be folded along crease line and hung from the cuffs on hangers with rubber-coated clips. Jeans, sweats and leggings should be folded and "filed" in drawers. If you have an abundance of shelf space, they can also be folded and stacked on shelves.

SHOES

There are many ways to store shoes, depending on the size and shape of your closet. If you are short on space, consider buying an under-the-bed shoe storage box, with separate compartments, and rotate shoes by the season. If we were perfect, we would use shoe trees in every single pair we own—Frank does, but he's a man and he's spoiled—or at the very least stuff them with tissue paper to retain shape. Most of us just toss shoes in a pile in the bottom of our closet—I'm guilty of this—so even putting them on a rack is an improvement. That's what I do now.

Try the following storage solutions:

✳ A telescoping low rack that holds two layers of shoes. It can be made as small or as long as it needs to be to fit. Fully extended, this type of rack will hold twenty pairs.

✳ A telescoping high rack. It's a taller version of the above, but it holds shoes in four layers. It's not as long, so will also hold about twenty pairs.

Closet Helpers

There are thousands of companies that offer closet organization services. Most will come to your home and make recommendations about rebuilding your closet space. They'll draw a floor plan and install fixtures for you. Expect to pay anywhere from about $200 to $2,000, depending on the size of your closet and the materials you select. The companies listed below have offices nationwide. Call the toll-free number to locate the store nearest you.

The California Closet Company
1–800–274–6745
The Closet Factory
1–800–692–5673

If you already have the right poles and shelving, browse through the following catalogs to find additional storage solutions. Call the toll-free number to order a catalog.

Lillian Vernon
1–800–285–5555
Hold Everything
1–800–421–2264

(Hold Everything also has twenty-seven stores in fourteen states. Call the above number to find the one closest to you.)

Also check out kitchen and bath stores for items that will work just as well in your closet. For example, a silverware tray is a terrific way to store jewelry, and stacking bath caddies work well for hose and socks. ✳

✳ Over-the-door shoe bag with pockets. This is usually plastic or canvas and holds each pair in a separate pocket. It can hold about twelve pairs.

✳ Custom-built shelves. You can place shoes alone, or in boxes (labeled) in a line. Holds as many pairs as you have space for. If you're going to do this, you really have to do it. Put shoes back in boxes after you wear them.

✳ If you have a special pair that you wear with only one outfit, hang it in a breathable fabric bag over the outfit's hanger.

✳ Sandals and athletic shoes can be stored in a basket.

SOCKS AND HOSE

These should be stored in a drawer, organizer caddy, or in mesh bags. The important thing is to organize them by color and type. Neatness counts here. Roll or fold socks and store them in a single layer. Hose stay safest when rolled. Do not store them in a drawer with a rough surface. Again, if socks or hose are worn with only one outfit, drape or hang them in a mesh bag with the outfit.

UNDERWEAR AND LINGERIE

Plastic bins in drawers work well to separate items (bra hooks can snag delicate panties). Over-the-door shoe bags are a great way to store individually. Also, this makes undergarments easily available while dressing. Hang special bras with the dress they belong with.

BELTS

Buy a round belt hanger—it works kind of like a key chain—to store all belts together. Never leave them in pants or skirts. You can also install a set of hooks on the back wall of a closet and hang belts by the buckle. That's what I've done in my closet. Or coil and place belts in a drawer.

SCARVES

Good scarves usually come with their own boxes. I recommend refolding and storing scarves in those boxes. For all others, either fold them neatly and place on shelves, or drape from hooks. If you use hooks, don't pack them in; they may get lost. Find a space that has a little room around it to keep scarves from wrinkling.

HANDBAGS

Storage depends on how often you use each type of bag. If most of your bags are the seasonal or special-occasion type, consider buying an under-the-bed storage box.

Stuff bags with tissue paper, fold soft handles inside, and snap shut. Place them in a box, or if you have the shelf space, line them up on a shelf (without cramming them in). Evening and smaller bags can be hung from hooks installed on the back wall of your closet.

COATS, GLOVES, BOOTS, AND OUTDOOR CLOTHING

These items should be stored in a separate closet close to your front door. Use the same criteria for cleaning out that closet and pitch damaged, missing (one glove), or outgrown articles. During the off season, stuff boots with wool gloves and scarves (toss in a few moth balls).

So there you have it, your closets and drawers are cleaned and organized. Now you can have that well-deserved bath. Enjoy that sundae. Rest up, because soon we are going to talk about what is missing from your closet. When we are done, you will have the basics to build on. Now aren't you glad you made all of that space?

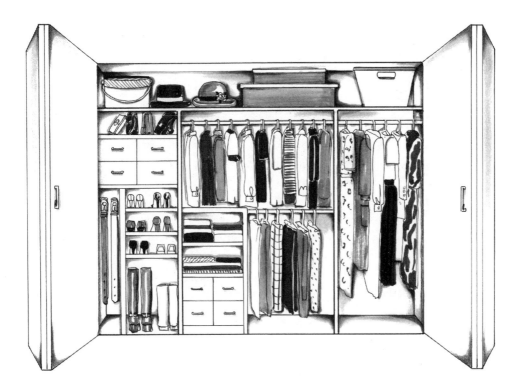

Chapter 3

Make More of Less
and Less of More

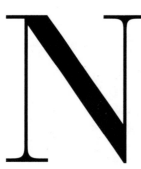obody's perfect. No body is either. We all have flaws in our figures that we wish we could deep-six. You can diet and exercise to change your figure somewhat, but short of extensive plastic surgery, there's not much you can do about your body's bone structure. And there's nothing you can do to change your height. What you can do is learn to dress in ways that emphasize your assets and hide your flaws.

As women, we throw around the word "hate" pretty freely. As in, "I just hate my hips." But often what we hate is a figment of our imagination. We're not nearly as unattractive as we think we are. Other people probably never see the blimp hips you think you have. Unless, of course, you wear clothes that accentuate the wrong parts. Tight leggings with a crop top broadcast, "Look at me, folks, I've got the biggest hips you've ever seen. And they're jiggly, too!"

With me, it's always been my thighs. Not my calves or my knees, but my thighs. When I was a teenager, I actually thought that people (boys) wouldn't like me because I had big thighs. I remember going to the beach with a group of girlfriends. They convinced me to wear a bathing suit, which I never did before. Of course, I also wore shorts over it to hide these enormous thighs. After a lot of teasing they finally persuaded me to remove the shorts. I remember thinking, *Oh no, no one's going to talk to me now.* But you know what? A group of boys came over and we talked and laughed all afternoon. No one stared at my legs or made rude comments. *They* didn't care what my thighs looked like. (I've since come to learn that men like the womanly attributes we hate the most. Go figure.) Like most people, they were so focused on themselves they didn't pay attention to such a trivial detail. So what did I learn? That the bad

perception of my thighs was my problem. I still don't like them, and I dress to cover them because it makes *me* happy. And that's the point. Make yourself happy. Learn to live with what you can't change and find ways to hide the stuff you don't want anyone else to see. It's all about you. No matter what you wear, you're still the same you underneath.

Look in the Mirror

To determine what you like and don't like about your body—you probably already know, but humor me—you will need to undress and stand in front of a full-length mirror. Keep all the weapons locked up and make sure there's nothing yummy to eat in the house, because if you're like me, you'll look in the mirror and run right to the kitchen. Now, assess yourself from head to toe. Would you like to look taller? Are your shoulders out of proportion with your hips? Breasts too small? Too large? Is your tummy a little larger than you'd like? Don't forget to use a hand-held mirror and peek at your back. You might think your bottom is too large or your hips are too wide. . . . Don't worry. . . . We all do. Once you identify your problem areas, consult the following pages to find the solutions that will improve your

An Emotional Makeover

Carol Luiken, a dresser on *All My Children,* called me and asked me to help her dress Jillian Spencer, who was then playing the character of Daisy. She was full-figured and hated her body. Carol had taken her to all the best stores, places like Bergdorf Goodman and Saks, to help her pick clothes that would emphasize her assets, but these excursions always dissolved into teary fights and Jillian's refusal to come out of the dressing room.

I invited her to my house, gave her a glass of wine, and asked her to strip to her undies so I could see her body. Of course, that brought tears, so I offered to show her my body to make her feel better. I grabbed a glass of wine for myself and stripped down. She cried, I cried, then she began to realize that if I could take my bumpy thighs and dress in such a way that no one knew I had them, then maybe she could dress that way, too.

We tried lots of outfits and finally came up with some that made her happy about the way she looked. It was all a matter of choosing styles that flattered her figure instead of pointing out its flaws. ✳

figure. These ideas won't change your body, but they will improve the way you look and what other people see. Shed your Sweatshopper ways, and you'll be happier with the way you look and feel. Again, let's work from the outside in. Once you see how great you can look, you may be inspired to hit the gym and tighten up those loose thighs once and for all.

To determine your body type, have someone take a full-length photograph of you. Stand straight with your arms at sides, with feet directly under hips. Use a marker to make a dot on each shoulder, on both sides of your waist, and on each hip. Connect the dots—across shoulders, down one side, across hips, and up to other shoulder—to see your shape.

Body Types

Later in this chapter are ideas for altering single body flaws like wide hips or narrow shoulders, but since most women have a number of areas they need to balance out, we need to concentrate on your body type first; then you can go to the sections that deal with single flaws for more ideas. On the following pages are the six most common body types and their fashion fixes. Remember, illusion is everything.

Pear-shaped

(Most of us are built this way.) Narrower shoulders than hips, defined waist, curvy hips and thighs, maybe a little tummy.

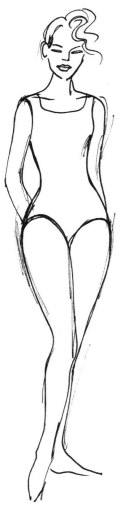

JACKET

You need to create the illusion of larger shoulders. Make sure jackets have small shoulder pads (not football-player huge). Jacket should be tailored and slightly (really, just slightly) flared to show off waist.

SKIRT

Skirt should be tapered in to create illusion of a slim line. Buy a straight skirt and have it taken in if needed. No A-lines for a pear-shaped figure.

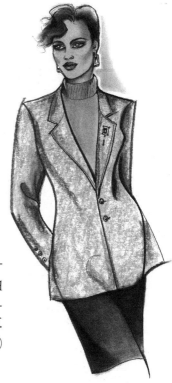

SLACKS

Never wear wide, flared slacks. They just call attention to the big bottom half. Buy fitted slacks (no pleats) with narrow legs.

Rectangle

Large and round from the shoulders to the hips, no defined waist, balanced on thinner legs.

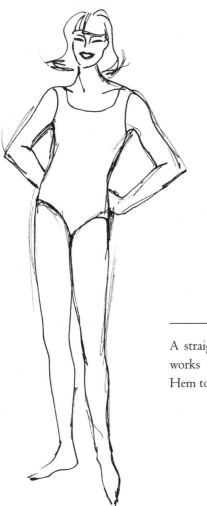

JACKET

A long four-button jacket is perfect for this figure. Small shoulder pads will create illusion of a thinner waist. Stay away from boxy or double-breasted styles. Keep lapels small.

SKIRT

A straight skirt—no belt—works best for a rectangle. Hem to just above knees.

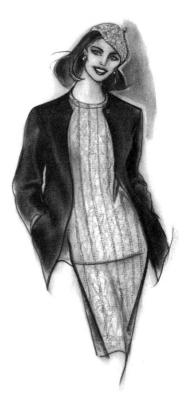

SLACKS

You want to create the illusion of length, not width, so wear straight, narrow slacks. Try not to tuck in shirts or wear big belts.

Hourglass

Balanced shoulders and hips, well-proportioned bust, defined waist.

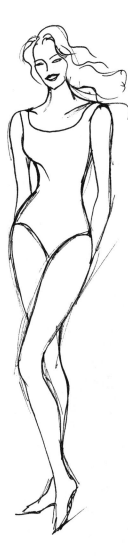

JACKET

This figure can wear just about any type jacket. A short jacket or a long one with a tailored waist are my favorites.

SKIRT

A long (ankle-length) skirt is a good choice.

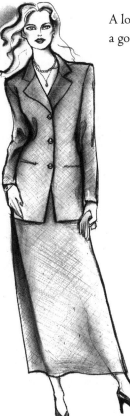

SLACKS

Either narrow- or wide-leg slacks look nice on an hourglass. If you don't have a large tummy, you can wear pleated slacks, too.

Triangle

Broader shoulders than hips, defined waist but straight hips, narrow pelvis, and flat bottom.

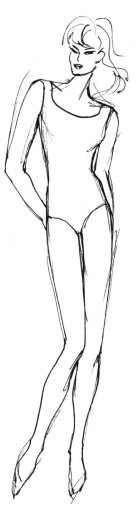

JACKET

———————————

Unconstructed, no shoulder pads, maybe belted at waist. Keep lapels narrow.

SKIRT

———————————

A flared or A-line skirt looks great on a triangle figure.

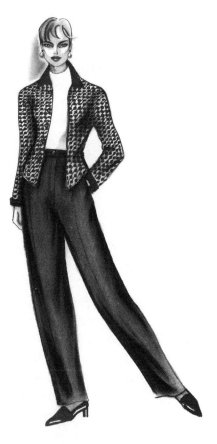

SLACKS

———————————

Pleated slacks will add illusion of wider hips to balance large shoulders.

Big Girl

Overly tall, proportioned figure, but big all over. Not necessarily fat.

JACKETS

Separates are made for big girls. A plaid jacket, with solid slacks, cuts height. Jacket must be long and narrow, with small lapels.

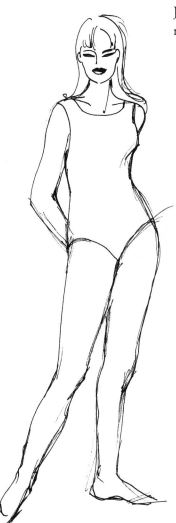

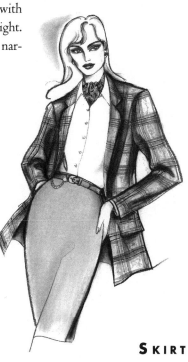

SKIRT

A straight skirt, hemmed two inches above knee, cuts height and slims.

SLACKS

Keep slacks plain and narrow. No pleats. Make sure they are long enough.

Petite and Round

Short, large waist and hips, shape not defined.

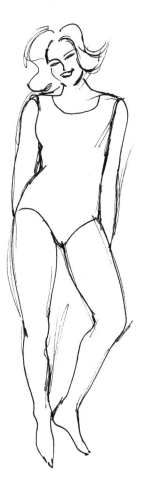

JACKET

———

Make sure jacket is right length (sleeves, too). Shop in the petite section or have clothes tailored. If you are round—large breasted, a bit of a tummy—don't wear boxy or double-breasted styles.

SKIRT

———

Wear skirts just above the knee. If tummy and bottom are round, wear straight styles.

SLACKS

———

Keep detail to a minimum. No pleats. Straight and narrow from hips to ankles.

Height

If you're five-three there's not much you can do to look five-ten, but there are tricks you can use to gain a couple of inches. Since looking taller also makes you look thinner you'll be killing two birds with one stone.

* Dress in one color from head to toe. Wear a jacket with either a skirt or pants in the same color, and then match your hose and shoes as closely as you can. Wear a blouse or shirt that is in the same color family but one or two shades lighter or darker.

* Wear a pantsuit—all one color—with narrow legs. Skinny trousers will lengthen leg.

* Wear your skirts an inch or two shorter—just above the knee is good. Showing a little more leg gives the illusion of length.

* Wear clothes that are fitted. Loose, boxy jackets will make you look wider, not taller.

* Choose a jacket length that falls just below the hip bone. Waist-length jackets will cut height.

* Wear vertical stripes. Not wide, bright ones, but subtle pin stripes on a jacket or blouse.

* Wear heels. But remember, spike heels on a small woman look ridiculous during the day. Instead, opt for a solid one-and-a-half-inch square heel. Rounded toes are more comfortable and create a softer look.

Arm Wrestling

About a year ago on *Another World,* Felicia had a formal party to attend that required a splashy evening gown. A week before we taped that show I went down to wardrobe for a fitting and just about fainted when I saw the red strapless gown meant for me. You already know that I have a thing about my thighs, but I also have a problem with showing my arms. I don't like them, I don't show them, and that's that.

I begged Lee, who was my wardrobe person, to allow me to wear a different dress. "Please, please," I said, "I'll do anything, just don't make me wear that dress." He didn't back down, and actually, everyone who came in said I looked wonderful, what was I talking about? I finally convinced him to let me wear a red shawl over my shoulders, but I became totally obsessed with wearing this getup. I couldn't concentrate on my acting. My lines were a big jumble in my head because all I was thinking about was positioning that damn shawl. I had to wear that dress for almost a week of taping and by the end I was a wreck. I didn't confide my feelings to anyone. I didn't say anything. I just loathed myself in quiet agony.

A few weeks later I was at home and turned on *World* for a minute, and—oh my God—there I was in that red dress! *Wait a minute,* I thought, *I don't look that bad. My arms look like normal arms.* Did I really just ruin a week of my life because I inflated the size of my arms in my head? What a moron! My reaction to wearing this dress was totally wrong and dumb, too. We do see ourselves differently from how others do, don't we? *

Shoulders
Too Wide

✳ These days it's hard to buy sweaters and blouses without shoulder pads, but that doesn't mean you have to wear them. Cut threads and remove them.

✳ Wear V-neck or scoop-neck tops to break up the width of shoulders.

✳ Don't wear square necklines; strapless tops or dresses; wide-scoop or boat-neck lines; or halter tops. They draw attention to shoulders and will make them look wider.

✳ Don't choose styles with any decoration on the shoulders. The military look is not for you.

✳ If your hips are small, don't wear tight skirts or pants, they will only make shoulders look more out of proportion.

Know Your Fit

Recently on *World,* my (former) dresser tried to make me wear an Ellen Tracy pink flared dress with a tiny little pink jacket over it, with black buttons. Now, I have a pear-shaped figure and I know it. I looked like an old, fat Nancy Reagan. I *know* I can't wear an A-line anything because it makes my hips and thighs look bigger than they are. This is one thing I'm really certain of (let's not even get into how I feel about pink!). My dresser kept insisting that I looked fine and should wear the outfit on the air. I'm rarely a prima donna on the set, but this time I stuck to my guns. There are some things you just know about your figure, and you can't let anyone else—your husband, a salesperson—convince you otherwise. ✳

Too Narrow

✳ Wear shoulder pads. If you have a shirt or jacket without them, buy extra pairs and sew a Velcro strip on pads and inside garment. They are easy to attach and to remove for washing.

✳ Wear tailored tops. Loose caftany-type things will make shoulders look formless and rounded.

✳ Choose styles that bare shoulders. Halters, strapless tops, and boat necks are all good for you.

✳ Don't wear anything that draws the eye to the center of your body. A large scarf or bulky necklace will make shoulders appear smaller.

Breasts
Too Small

✳ Wear a push-up or padded bra when the style calls for cleavage. (For a complete review of undergarments, see Chapter 9: Under It All.)

✳ Wear styles that cut the body line. Waist-length sweaters or jackets add bulk to the chest area. Tuck shirts in.

✳ Wear heart-shaped or round necklines. Higher necklines flatten you out.

✳ Thicker fabrics will pump you up. Angora or mohair sweaters look great on small-breasted women.

✳ Wear layers, such as a blouse, then a vest, then a jacket, to give the illusion of substance.

✳ Choose tops with pockets or decorations over chest area.

✳ Wear a wide cinch belt with a dress to cut vertical lines.

✳ Wear scarves and bulky necklaces as your final layer.

Too Large

✳ Wear solid-color shirts and jackets. Prints, stripes, and patterns draw attention to the breasts and designs look stretched.

✳ Wear navy, black, or brown on top. Lighter colors make breasts appear larger.

✳ Wear dresses that have an A-line or drop waist.

Good Times I've Missed

Years ago, Frank, who worked in advertising, had Club Med as an account. We were always being invited to tour their many resorts, and I always refused. I saw the ads for these clubs: I saw those beautiful, tight-muscled European women and said—no, shouted—"No way!" I wasn't going to sunbathe in public next to these perfect bodies. Absolutely not!

Then one day when we were in the Bahamas, Frank had to meet his client at the Club Med there and insisted I come along. I did. Fully clothed. Well, I looked around and saw lots of different types of women, all of whom were relaxed and enjoying themselves. Some *were* gorgeous, but most were average. I kicked myself. *I could have come here,* I thought. Why do I deny myself pleasure, keep myself from experiencing fun things, because of my hangups about my body? Why do I always do without? It's so silly. *I'm silly.* But no more. I deserve to do fun things and so do you. Please, don't give up a great experience just because you're worried about your appearance. I guarantee, no one is going to notice how you look; we're all too hung up on how we look to worry about your big tushy. ✳

* Don't wear double-breasted jackets. Choose single-breasted, one-button styles that can be left open.

* Stick with simple styles. Avoid pockets and appliqués.

* Wear open collars or V-necks that fit. If your breasts are spilling out the top, you'll only draw attention to them.

* Wear wide-leg pants to balance proportions.

* Wear big, chunky heels. They'll help lengthen the body and divert attention from breasts.

* Wear earrings to draw eye up and away from breasts.

* Don't wear a wide belt or tuck a tight shirt into pants.

* Wear the right size support bra with wide, comfortable shoulder straps.

Waist
Too Small

* Boy, are you lucky. Still, sometimes a small waist will make hips appear bigger. To avoid, don't cinch belts too tight, or wear skirts or pants that have pleats that fall on hips.

Too Wide

* Try not to wear belts at all. If you cinch them too tight, skin (or fat) will hang over the top and look unflattering. If you leave them loose, they won't change anything.

* Wear dresses that have a drop waist or are A-line. A loose sheath dress works well because it hangs on hips and you can't really see the waist.

* Draw attention away from your waist and to the legs by wearing shorter skirts. A long, full skirt will do the same thing.

* Wear scarves and earrings to draw eye up and away from waist.

* Wear pants with elastic or simple waistbands.

* Wear tops that cover waist. Loose tunics and wrap styles work well. A long vest also does the trick.

* Wear tops with shoulder pads to even out proportions.

Short-Waisted

* Dress in one color to lengthen body.

* Wear jackets, shirts, and vests that fall below the waistline.

* Don't tuck in blouses tightly. Let some fabric fall over waistband.

* Wear high-necked tops to create illusion of length.

* Don't wear high-waisted slacks or skirts. Choose styles that rest on hips instead.

* Wear belts draped around hips, not cinched tightly around waist.

Long-Waisted

* Wear separates in different colors to break up length of body.

* Wear jackets, shirts, and vests that fall near waistline.

* Don't wear long tops that are fitted. Choose looser styles that cover waistline instead.

* Wear strapless or deep scoop-neck tops to break up your body and make it look shorter.

* Wear high-waisted slacks or skirts. Hip huggers will just make your body look even longer.

* Wear the right length pants. Hem should break over the top of your shoe. And don't wear pants with cuffs; they will make your legs look shorter.

* Wear plain belts. Otherwise you'll draw attention to a long waist.

Legs
Too Short

❋ Don't wear wide-leg pants, or those with heavy pleats or cuffs.

❋ Wear shorter skirts; they will add length to legs.

❋ Wear stirrup pants or other pants with long narrow legs.

❋ Wear cropped or waist-length tops; they create the illusion of longer legs.

❋ Wear short jackets, such as a peplum style.

❋ Don't wear ankle-high boots; they cut legs off.

Too Long

This is only a problem if your waist is short, or if your legs are super skinny, making you look unbalanced. To correct:

❋ Wear wide-leg, or harem pants. Cropped pants also work well.

❋ Wear mid-length (between knee and ankle) skirts to break up length.

❋ Wear jackets that come to about mid-thigh.

❋ Wear boots to ankle or just under knee. Don't wear thigh-huggers; they'll only make legs look longer.

❋ Wear contrasting-color hose, but not patterned.

Too Thick

❋ Don't wear tapered pants. Opt for wide-leg pants with little detail instead. Pajama-style or palazzo pants in a fabric that drapes easily work well.

❋ Don't wear heavily pleated pants or those with large pockets. They just add bulk that you don't need.

❋ Wear darker colors such as black, navy, or brown from the waist down. Always match hose to skirts to create a leaner look.

* Wear brighter colors from waist up to divert attention from thighs.

* Stay away from narrow, fitted skirts. Choose looser, longer styles instead.

* Don't wear jackets that stop at the waist or are fitted around thighs. Longer, looser styles will cover thighs smoothly.

* Wear support undergarments that hold thighs in (see Chapter 9: Under It All).

* Wear shoes that will support your weight, but are not too chunky. Spike heels are not good, but neither are thick, lug-soled loafers. A solid one-inch heel in a feminine style works best.

Hips
Too Wide

* Wear tops with shoulder pads to even out proportions.

* Wear long, untucked blouses or vests that cover hips.

* Don't wear short jackets; they will emphasize hips.

* Wear straight-styled dresses (ones that fall from the shoulder) that do not require a belt. Dresses are the best weapon against this problem, so find a few you like and stick with them.

* Wear pants with slight pleats in front to balance out width.

* Wear pants with pockets on side seams so you don't add bulk to hips.

Bottom
Too Large

* Wear darker colors below the waist, lighter above.

* Wear jackets and vests that cover your bottom. A really long vest, one that matches your dress or skirt hemline, works best.

✳ Wear single-button jackets that are not tightly fitted around your bottom.

✳ Wear wide-leg pants, which will not show the difference between your bottom and thighs as profoundly.

✳ Don't wear pants or skirts with pockets on the rear.

✳ Wear loose or draped skirts. Stay away from tight fabrics like Lycra or Spandex.

✳ Don't wear leggings unless your top completely covers your rear.

Too Flat

✳ Wear long jackets or vests to cover bottom, or choose styles that flair out from the waist and drape over your bottom to add extra bulk.

✳ Wear skirts and pants that have side pockets (back pockets will only call more attention to your flat tushy) and pleats to add depth.

✳ Wear belts to create the illusion of more shape below the waist.

✳ Wear padded underwear (for a full review, see Chapter 9: Under It All).

Flabby Stomach

✳ Wear jackets and vests that are loose and cover the stomach.

✳ Wear dresses with an Empire (high) waistline. Fabric will fall from under the breasts and cover your stomach.

✳ Don't wear tight pants or skirts. Choose styles that are roomy in front, but not pleated.

✳ Wear skirts and pants with side or back zippers to avoid adding more bulk in front.

❋ Make sure pants have the right length rise (length from crotch to waist) for you. Nothing looks worse than pants that are bunched up and tight in the crotch area; the eye will be drawn to the area you're trying to hide.

❋ Wear tummy-flattening support panties.

Thick Calves and Ankles

❋ Don't wear cropped or tight pants.

❋ Wear long skirts that fall loosely. Miniskirts will highlight thick lower legs.

❋ Do wear boots. Those that come to just below the knee solve this problem nicely.

❋ Don't wear shoes that have details—such as straps—around the ankle.

❋ Wear medium-height heels to lengthen legs, but don't go overboard and wear too-tall heels; they'll make your legs look too heavy for the shoes.

Big All Over

❋ The trick for larger women is to find clothes that are loose enough to cover flaws, yet still look tailored and neat. Clothes that are too large and baggy will only draw attention to weight.

❋ Wear darker colors from head to toe. Add color with accessories.

❋ Wear clothes made from quality fabrics that will hold their shape. Choose light-weight fabrics—so you don't add bulk—with a tight weave.

❋ If most of your weight is above the legs, wear narrow-leg pants with medium-height heels.

❋ Wear single-button (button at the neck) jackets and vests that fall easily over stomach and hips.

❋ Don't tuck in tops.

✳ Wear dresses that are tailored around shoulders and fall more loosely over body. Shirt or coat dresses work well.

✳ Add a waistline with a loosely buckled belt.

✳ Wear jewelry—but not too much. Earrings and a simple, long necklace draw the eye up to the face and away from the body. Don't heap on necklaces, though; they add bulk.

✳ Do investigate support undergarments to streamline your figure (see Chapter 9: Under It All).

Chapter 4

———

Let's Go Shopping

I have to be honest. I love shopping. I love it to the point that I might even have a spending disorder. If I'm feeling fat or unloved, or unappreciated or nuts about anything, I'll go shopping. I know it sounds silly, but I love everything about it. Looking at pretty things, touching them, thinking about wearing them, crowds, sales, finding the bargain of a lifetime. For me, the search is more fun than the conquest.

I also like shopping because it's social. Not necessarily because I go with a group of friends—I'm generally a loner—but because I like to talk to strangers about fabrics and fit and anything to do with clothes. If you see me out shopping, feel free to come up and say hello. We'll talk. I'll tell you what I think. We might even have lunch if I have the time. The social part of shopping is huge for me. It certainly brought my mother and I together. It's a love we share. Maybe that's where it all began; my mother, like me, loves to shop.

Having admitted to this obsession, as much as I *like* shopping, even I have to remember that it has a purpose. If I allow myself to wander aimlessly through stores, not looking for anything in particular, I undoubtedly will end up buying something I don't need and can't wear. Now, not everyone likes shopping. You may hate it. If you hate it, treat it like a job. You're not well enough trained to treat it casually. Not yet, anyway.

The way I tackle my inclination to window shop (which always leads to impulsive buying) is to make lists. I simply can't remember the details of everything I need, so I write them down. I use my appointment book. An entry may look something like this: black belt with gold-tone buckle (Okay, so it's just gold, but the fashion types always say gold-tone) to go with black suit-dress. If I don't write it down, here's what will happen: I'll be in a store and think, *Oh yeah, I need a belt. Now what color is it I need? I think I need a black belt.* So I buy a black belt with a great silver-tone buckle. Then I get home and realize that not only will the silver buckle clash with the gold buttons on my dress, but I already have another belt exactly like the one I just bought! I put the new belt in a bag and promise myself to return it and get the right belt. But you know what? I never do. I can't remember. This is why I write this stuff down and why you should, too.

Writing things down is only one of the many unbreakable rules for shopping that I have developed over the years. Read on for the rest of my treasured secrets.

Top Ten Rules for Shopping Wisely

1.   Know What You Need

You know what your fashion weaknesses are, you've cleaned out and reorganized your closet, and all the clothes in it now are ones that fit and are in good shape. So what is missing from your wardrobe that will really pull it together? This is where most women get into trouble. You think if you don't buy something flashy, no one will notice you. You don't think about what your wardrobe needs are; you think about some image in your head. Who wants to buy a plain white shirt? You do, if you don't have this most basic item. So now is the time to make your first list. It may be just a wish list. You may not be able to afford everything you write down, but do it anyway. You need to be able to see a clear path to where you and your wardrobe are going. Carry this list with you when you go shopping.

2.   Make a Budget for the Season (and Stick to It)

Decide how much you can spend this season to upgrade your wardrobe. This is really important. If you have $500 to spend, you have to figure out which items will add the most punch to things you already own. I have never had a client who had to start completely from scratch and I doubt you will have to, either. Compare your budget with your wish list and rearrange the list in priority order. If you can only afford the first ten items on your list, then buy only those items. There's always next season. The things you carefully buy now will last forever, so don't become overanxious and try to get everything right away. Oh, and don't buy anything with your precious budgeted money that's not on your list. You can't. Not yet.

3. Dress the Part

If you're looking for the perfect buttercup-yellow blouse to go with your brown suit, wear the suit while shopping. It's the only way to get a perfect match and to check the fit. You might get the color right, but the collar may look awful with the jacket. Also, salespeople will be better able to help you find what you're looking for if you bring along or wear the clothes you are trying to augment.

Another reason (okay, two reasons) to dress well when you shop is that it will make you feel prettier and more confident about yourself. You cannot look pretty in a new suit if you are not wearing the right hose or shoes. If your hair is dirty, everything will look off. You must wear makeup. Don't go shopping if you can't pull yourself together for the trip. And, this is the truth, you'll get more help from salespeople. They'll see that you are serious about finding—and buying—the right item.

4. Take a Friend

None of us are objective about how we look. A friend—she has to be honest and have good taste—will see you from all angles, including the rear. She'll tell you that those slacks make your bottom look like a blimp. She'll also be able to run back and forth from the dressing room to the floor to find you the right sizes so you don't have to keep getting dressed over and over again. I'm allowed to shop alone because I'm good at it, but you can't unless you read this entire book and practice until you get it right.

5. Give Yourself Enough Time

Never, ever shop on Saturday morning for the dress you need on Saturday night. You'll spend too much and buy the wrong thing. If you find the perfect dress, but it's a little long, you won't have time to get it tailored. So you'll wear it long, and look and feel crummy. If your feet hurt, if your back hurts, if you're tired, go home. Come back another day. You can't make good decisions if you're feeling awful, and you'll buy all kinds of things that are wrong, wrong, wrong.

6. Ask About Services

As soon as you enter the store, ask if they have a personal shopper and an alterations department. If a personal shopper is not available, snag a salesperson and tell her your needs. Let her know that you expect her to stay with you until you've found what you're looking for. Many stores have cut back on salespeople, and they can be hard to find. If you're nice and direct with them—"I really need your advice, can you help me?"—they will respond.

If you find something you love that sort of fits, go directly to the store tailor. Right then, that day. Don't leave the store until you do (often they can do alterations while you shop). If I see you on the street with your jacket sleeves rolled up and you're holding this book, I'll come over and smack you with it. You have to focus on the details. They are what will make you appear well-dressed.

Where the Deals Are

You can find bargains on TV, but you have to learn how to recognize them. I have found that the best buys are in jewelry, handbags, and other accessories. I once bought a backpack from QVC that sold in a store on Madison Avenue in New York City for much more. I probably wouldn't have bought it if I hadn't known its real value. So, go ahead, browse expensive boutiques and department stores to learn about quality and price. Note brand names that you really like. When they show up on TV for less money, go for it. ✳

7. Accessorize

You've bought the outfit, now what? Don't you leave the store without stopping in the scarf and jewelry departments. You may not buy anything today, but check it out. See what you might wear to add some pizzazz to your purchase. Buy the hose or socks you need. You have the outfit right there, what better time to match the color? Last, stroll through the shoe department. Is there a special pair of shoes that adds just that little bit of style you need? Maybe not, but look anyway.

8. Try on Everything

I used to stay away from high-priced designer departments because I knew I couldn't afford the clothes. But that was stupid. You know why? Because I was limiting myself. What I've discovered is that certain designers fit me really well. I might find a perfect jacket that is way out of my price range. I could pass it over because I don't want to blow my whole budget on one item, or I could buy it and turn it into a real wardrobe winner. How? I take the jacket to a tailor and have it copied. I've bought a $600 designer jacket (I can't tell you which designer or they will write me nasty letters) and had it copied for $160. Yes, $600 is a lot, but I can now have that jacket copied over and over for the rest of my life in any fabric I choose. That and the fact that it fits me like a glove make the price worth it.

The other reason to head for the designer departments is so that you can learn about quality and fit. You need to touch the fabrics, examine the stitching, and try on the very best clothes so that later, when you're sifting through the outlet racks, you can identify quality. It's almost like being a student and studying for a test. Learn to identify the good stuff—even though you can't afford it—and you'll pass with flying colors.

The Outlet Trap

I went to Woodbury Commons, an outlet mall about an hour and a half from my house, for a day of shopping. I walked that mall from end to end and really didn't see anything I loved. But I had come so far! I had to buy something. I ended up buying a designer blazer that wasn't even a great bargain. Now, usually I love this designer and her other clothes have always fit me quite well. This blazer didn't. Every time I wear it, I'm tugging and pulling, trying to get it to work. I never feel comfortable in it. I think I still try to wear it because I feel so guilty about breaking my own rule—I don't love this blazer. So now I'm doubling my mistake. I never should have bought it in the first place. Oh well, I learned my lesson. ✳

9. Keep Your Eyes Open

I can't tell you how many times I have tried on an outfit that fit perfectly and looked great but that I didn't buy. Why didn't I buy it? Well, I did—just not all of it. I'll try on a jacket and skirt that is made to go with a blouse from the same designer. Maybe the blouse is a little black T-shirt–like thing that sells for $80. It does really complete the suit, but it's eighty bucks! I know that the little store down the street always stocks basic tops in every color and they're only $20. How do I know this? Because when I shop, I also scout the stores and make a mental note of what they carry for just this scenario. Now, if given the choice, would you spend $80 for the designer T-shirt, or $20 for the exact same thing down the street? Good girl, I knew you'd make the right choice. By the way, this only works if you actually go to the other store and buy the shirt. Do it right away, before you get home and stow the suit in the back of your closet because you have nothing to wear with it.

10.   You Gotta Love It

Whatever you buy, you must love it. It has to make you sing. If I have to ask a friend—now remember, I'm good at this—if they like it, I won't buy it. I know *I* have to love it. If my friend likes it so much, I'll let her buy it. You know you've graduated when you can shop alone and not second-guess yourself.

The Fitting-Room Survival Guide

I can't think of any place I'd rather avoid than a fitting room. Many other women feel the same way. I think that's why catalogs and TV-shopping channels have enjoyed so much success. Even though it's a hassle to return things that don't fit, it's more comforting to try on clothes at home. We'd all rather have root canal than try on a bathing suit at Macy's (or any other store). Am I right? And forget about stores that have a communal dressing room. I didn't take showers after gym class in junior high, and I'm not going to start undressing in front of strangers now. Especially now. Not only do people look at me because I'm Felicia Gallant, but they're shocked when I don't live up to their perfect expectations.

I don't really understand why, if it's the goal of stores to sell clothes, they don't do everything possible to make the fitting rooms as clean and flattering to customers as possible. Why the fluorescent lighting? Why doors that only hide you from the knees to the shoulders? Why have no mirrors in the room itself, forcing you to step outside to see how you look? Your guess is as good as mine.

So how to combat dressing-room hell? Well, for one thing—and I've mentioned this before—always wear makeup when you shop. At the very least, bring a tube of lipstick so you won't look dead. If your face is bare there is no way you will look attractive under those lights. Your natural skin tone will look green and clash with

The Catalog Trap

My dear friend Barbara has what I call a return disorder. She orders excessively from catalogs. She views it like getting a gift. The mail carrier, who knows her personally by now, arrives every day with a new box. *Oh, a gift for me!* she thinks. Even though she ordered it and knows what's inside, she still reacts like it's Christmas every day. The problem is, she orders things she can't or won't wear. Then she doesn't return anything—ever. She throws it away! This is *my* friend, who knows all the rules, who does this! I haven't been able to break her of this expensive and destructive habit, so I just tease her about it. You, however, have to return unwanted items. Right away. I don't want you to fall into the same trap as Barbara. ✳

whatever color you are trying on. If you're concerned about getting makeup on the clothes, ask for a face shield. The better stores stock them; they're soft paper shields that snap around your neck to protect clothes.

Carry a brush or comb in your purse. Fix hair after you put on an outfit and *before* you look in the mirror. If you often wear your hair back or up, wear it that way to shop so it will stay neater when trying on clothes.

Wear tights or pantyhose. If I tried on a dress without hose, I wouldn't be inspired to run to the gym and work off that cellulite; I'd head straight to the coffee bar and eat six doughnuts. So give yourself a fair chance and make sure your legs are properly outfitted before trying on a dress or suit. Swimsuits are a whole different story. There's really nowhere to hide. Nonetheless, I still wear pantyhose when trying them on. It's more sanitary and if I had to actually look at my legs under those lights . . . well . . . you know . . . ten doughnuts later I still wouldn't have a suit.

The mirrors in dressing rooms have a life all their own. The mirrors may be thinner that those at home and can distort the way you look. They also rarely reach the floor. Is there a conspiracy to keep us from seeing how we look from head to toe? I don't know what's going on there, but this is one of the best reasons to shop with a friend. They'll be more honest than the mirrors.

Personal Shoppers

A friend of mine was looking for a new basic suit—a basic, classic, simple kind of suit—and didn't know where to begin. Since I was doing this book, and because I have had only good experiences with personal shoppers, I wanted to know more about how the average person might use one. I talked my friend into doing a little research for me. I can't go myself because I get *too* much attention. I wanted to really know how you would be treated if you called a department store and asked for help. My friend called Nordstrom's and made an appointment. Over the phone, she told the shopper what she was looking for, her budget, and her size. She decided she had only $350 dollars to spend, and she hoped to get shoes included in that price, too. That might sound like a lot of money to some of you, but remember, this was to be the basic suit that would last forever.

My friend arrived at the store and went to the special office where the shoppers work with clients. It was a lovely area with a private dressing room. The shopper had selected a group of suits, all in the right size, all with matching blouses. My friend didn't see anything she really loved, so they headed out to the sales floor. The shopper knew every item in the store and was able to steer my friend to the departments that displayed suits in her price range.

They settled on a light-brown Eileen Fisher suit that came in at about $280 for the jacket and skirt. It was made to go with a simple blouse that cost $110. My friend, having scouted the stores, decided to skip the blouse, knowing she could get it for less than $30 elsewhere. Here's what happened next, the best part of this experience: She still needed shoes and had only $40 left in her budget after deducting $30 for the blouse. The personal shopper ran down to the shoe department and brought back the perfect pair of Adrienne Vittadini suede pumps. The color matched exactly. My friend loved these shoes. Even though they were $100 she decided to buy them. The only problem was that they didn't have her size. The shopper then turned on the computer and searched every Nordstrom's store in the country, but no luck, no one had the shoes. What happened next is the best reason ever to use a personal shopper. This one called *Bloomingdale's* to see if they had those shoes in my friend's size! She actually called another store. She took the time because even she agreed they were the perfect shoes. She didn't have to do it, she might have even gotten in trouble if her boss found out, but she wanted to really help my friend. Not only did Bloomingdale's have the shoes, they were on sale for $50 and they agreed to ship them directly to my friend's home. How's that for a deal? As if that weren't enough, the shopper dashed to the hosiery department and came back with two pair of matching hose, which my friend bought.

My friend ended up with exactly what she set out to find, for exactly the right price. She got a complete outfit, which she loves and feels great in, in less than two hours. Of course, she could have found this stuff herself, eventually (it may have taken weeks to track down the shoes), but as she said, "I got the benefit of the shopper's expertise and ability to coordinate this outfit. If I were alone, I probably would have given up. Also, I never felt, for a minute, that the shopper wasn't devoted to me just because I didn't have thousands of dollars to spend. This shopper has made a loyal customer out of me, for life."

Beware of Imitations

I was in Loehmann's in California a while ago and saw a whole rack of Bill Blass skirts. There must have been fifty of them. The designer label compelled me to look them over. The label did say Bill Blass, but the skirts were not his usual quality. The seams were loose, the style was a little weird. I thought, *How could this be?* An employee standing next to me must have read my mind, because she came over and told me that the fabric was indeed from Bill Blass. They had bought it from him (left over from a previous collection) and had someone else make up the skirts. If I weren't so well trained in identifying quality, I may have been duped, as I'm sure many other shoppers were. You have to know what you're buying—that's why I urge you to try on good clothes even if you can't afford to buy them. You need to learn. ✳

Not only did my friend get a great outfit, she made a connection with a fashion expert whom she knows she can rely on. The shopper now sends her news of upcoming sales and special events. My friend can call and ask her if the store carries something she is looking for—boy, does that save time.

I absolutely encourage you to try using a personal shopper until you learn how to shop alone. They truly want to, and can, help you. It's their job and they want to succeed for themselves as well as for you. Every major department store now employs them; all you have to do is call and make an appointment. Tell them what you are looking for, how much you can spend, and your sizes. They are especially helpful to larger-size women because they know which designers make bigger-style clothes. This will save you from running from department to department seeking the size you need. Also, I've just learned that malls now use personal shoppers. You can call them with a request, and they will search the entire mall for you. How's that for a time-saver?

Personal shoppers generally are not paid on commission so you don't have to feel obligated to buy anything unless you love it. They will be that friend you need to give advice on fit and style. They'll tell you how you look from behind. The only thing you have to do is make it clear that you want them to be honest with you. You have to let them know you can take criticism and will take their advice. If they know you value their opinion they can be the most helpful shopping friend you've ever had.

It's on Sale!

I bet you didn't realize that certain things always go on sale at the same time every year. It took me a while to figure it out, too, but since I have, it has made finding real bargains easier. I know when to wait a few weeks for a better buy and also when to expect to pay full price (sometimes you have to have that special something right away). Just before a season starts is often the best time to shop. Not only will you hit pre-season sales, you'll get stuff that is up-to-date and wearable right away. Use the chart on the following page as a guide to finding the best prices year-round.

JANUARY	FEBRUARY	MARCH	APRIL	MAY	JUNE
real and fake furs, winter coats, gloves, hats, scarves, cashmere and other high-quality sweaters	gold, diamonds, and other fine jewelry, snow boots, winter shoes, cashmere and other high-quality sweaters (now at clearance prices)	spring suits and separates (linens, light cottons, etc.), spring coats, raincoats, handbags, and wallets	raincoats (now at clearance prices), dressy separates (silks, satins), silk blouses, spring dresses	spring shoes, all spring suits and dresses (now at clearance prices)	swimwear (suits, coverups, etc.), shorts, summer casual shirts, summer dresses

JULY	AUGUST	SEPTEMBER	OCTOBER	NOVEMBER	DECEMBER
swimwear, shorts, summer casual shirts, summer shoes and sandals	clearance on all swimwear and summer sportswear, shoes (biggest shoe sale of the year), fall suits, fall dresses	wool suits, better raincoats, back-to-school sales, handbags, wallets, backpacks, trendy items	fall suits, winter coats, raincoats (now at clearance prices), leather jackets and pants, sporty sweaters	fall shoes, fall boots, winter coats and jackets, evening wear, sweaters	coats (now at clearance prices), gift sweaters (like cashmere or silk blends), gold, diamonds, and other fine jewelry, some evening wear

Outlet Shopping

Outlets or designer discount stores come in a variety of shapes and sizes. They range from freestanding stores like Loehmann's, Daffy's, T. J. Maxx, and The Dress Barn to huge outlet malls with hundreds of single shops. They are all very different in the type of merchandise they carry and how deep the discounts go. At Loehmann's—which is truly my second home—you will find leftovers from every designer and department store in the country. Although the selection is diverse, Loehmann's is not big on display and prettying up the clothes. You have to pick through racks crammed with clothes to find the great styles and bargains. It's very hit-or-miss: You may go on Monday and find nothing; on Tuesday there will be a treasure trove.

You will find a totally different experience at the outlet malls. These designer stores are generally very attractive and look no different from a regular retail store. Each store carries only one brand name (smaller designers often band together to open one store among them), although they will carry all of the designer's merchandise from the high-priced couture clothes to the cheaper bridge, or mass market, lines.

When these big malls first opened, wow!, what a deal they were. Not many people knew about them and the merchandise selection was terrific. Items may have been off-season, but they were still high quality and at wonderful prices. Clothes were the real thing: designer styles, top quality, too good to be true. However, things have changed at outlets, and I'm here to tell you, watch out. Outlets can be a minefield for an inexperienced shopper. Here's why: Many designers—but not all, that's why it's so confusing unless you know what you're doing—now make clothes exclusively for their outlet stores, compromising on quality and workmanship to sell at a lower price. These clothes never see retail stores at all; they are shipped directly to the outlet and may or may not even resemble the designer's real styles. The other reason to use caution is that the prices may not be that great. Outlets may offer a 30 percent discount off the supposed retail price, but you may do better shopping the sales at stores closer to home. Many end-of-season sales offer discounts of 50 percent or more.

So when you go to an outlet store, or Loehmann's, or Filene's Basement, you still have to follow your shopping rules to avoid mistakes. Don't enter without clutching your need-to-buy list in your hand and don't buy anything that's not on that list. No matter what. I know, I know, you went all that way to shop, you just have to buy something, right? Well, okay, you can buy a belt, or a scarf, maybe a handbag, but that's it unless you find something you absolutely love. I'd rather see you pay full retail price for that one amazing jacket than blow $500 on five shabby ones. You'll wear that expensive jacket every day and love how you look. The shabby ones? They'll be in your next pile of giveaways.

Before you buy anything at an outlet, inquire about their return policy. They may allow no returns or restrict them to seven days. If you are shopping far from home, this could be a problem. Will you really drive two hours to return something or will you just live with your mistake? Also, you may only be offered store credit. Will you come back and use the credit? Think it over before you buy.

So, shop outlets carefully. If you do find that great dress at half off? I'm thrilled for you. How lucky you are. Buy it and love it. I can't wait to see you in it!

Catalog Shopping/TV Shopping

I think—no I'm sure—that the main reason catalogs and television shopping have become so popular is that many women do not want to try on clothes in public. You may be uncomfortable with your size or having anyone see you undress, so you rely on mail- or phone-order fashion so you won't be embarrassed. You may also use catalogs because you're just too busy to shop. (You can save loads of time using a store personal shopper.) That's all okay if you know what you're doing; if you're ordering clothes you actually wear; if you're returning clothes you don't like or that don't fit. But if you're just ordering more of the same clothes you already own and stashing mistakes in the bottom of your closet, you're wasting money and not doing a thing toward building a wardrobe.

That's not to say that you can't find great deals on TV or in catalogs; you just have to be selective. When I came to QVC I promised them I could design Bergdorf's-style clothes at Kmart prices. And I have. I also haven't forgotten my large-size customers; all my designs come in 1X, 2X, and 3X. I don't just take little clothes and make them bigger; I design clothes that flatter the big body parts we hate most: hips and thighs. When you shop on my show, I can promise you, you will find clothes that not only make you feel terrific but are priced right and go with other clothes you already own.

But I'm not the only designer selling clothes on TV. How do you know what you are getting? You have to listen to the host describe the item. They will usually tell you about the fabric, how it launders and how well it wears. TV hosts will tell you the truth because they want to minimize returns. Also, most stations have a strict quality-control office that edits out duds. Watch how the models wear the clothes. What else are they wearing with an item? How are they accessorizing it? If you decide to order, it's okay to ask the phone operator questions. Ask them to restate the fabric content. Does it run large or small? Most important, what is the return policy? How much time do you have to return? Will they pay postage? Most TV shopping shows will take back any item without a reason. Not liking something is a good enough reason.

You really can't beat the convenience of shopping from your living room, but can you find quality clothes at good prices? You can, but you have to follow the same shopping rules you would in a store (it's easy to get sucked in from the comfort of your couch). Keep your need-to-buy list right next to the remote control, and don't pick up the phone unless the item is on your list and you love it. If you do buy something, try it on as soon as it arrives. If you love it, but the fit is a little off, take it to a tailor right away. Don't wait, and don't wear it until it's fixed. If it isn't really what you expected, repack it and return it now. Don't put it on a chair or in your closet; return it while it's right there in your hand and you still have the packing materials.

The safest buy in TV shopping is accessories. You don't have to worry about how they'll fit, and the models on the air will show you how to wear them. Buy a scarf, a pin, a hat, a belt, or a handbag. Many are one-of-a-kind items, designed specifically for the TV sale, so you'll be getting a unique accessory that you can wear right away, no matter how big your thighs are. As for price on TV shopping shows, you have to do your homework. That's why I always say to scout the stores when you're shopping. Not necessarily to buy, but so you'll recognize a bargain when you see one.

Catalog shopping can be good and bad. Good because it's convenient and you can get a lot of basics without leaving home; bad because you can't really see the fabric and the way it moves. I use catalogs to buy basics like turtlenecks and other simple shirts, which I'll wear under a jacket or vest. I also buy socks and specialty items like outerwear (ski jackets, hats, gloves). I also order jewelry—not the expensive stuff, I leave that to Frank—from catalogs because I can often find one-of-a-kind items. What I don't order are slacks or dresses because they require a more specific fit. I need to try on fifty pairs of slacks before I'll buy one. What you can do is order a few different styles (check the return policy), try them on and return those that don't work for you. If, by some miracle, you do find a pair that fit and feel great, consider ordering another pair in a different color. You've hit the gold mine and shouldn't pass it by. You may find that one catalog carries items that always fit you well. If you do, hang on to it, because that means they cut their clothes in a way that works for you. If one item fits well, chances are all the items in that catalog are sized right for you.

Catalogs, like stores, have sales. They are usually just before a season starts, or for real bargains, right after a season ends. To successfully shop catalogs, you have to keep a pile of them. I have a stack, which I edit every time a new one comes in the mail. The new season comes, I toss the old one. If you don't do this you'll end up with two hundred catalogs and never be able to find the one you need. So, back to sales. At the end of a season, a sale catalog will arrive—often it's a section of the next season's catalog. If the sale includes your basics—a white shirt, a black sweater—by all means, buy it and keep it for next year (just remember where you stored it).

If you'd like to receive more catalogs, all you have to do is call the 800 directory (800-555-1212, it's free) and ask for the number of the company whose catalog you'd like to receive. Call them, and believe me, they will be more than happy to send you a copy.

TV Shopping Lesson

One of the things that TV shopping channels do is sell an item until it's gone. They can't return items because many are made especially for that show and have no retail outlet. If it's in their warehouse, they're gonna try and sell it. Unless you watch regularly, there's no way for you to know that you're seeing an item that they have been trying to get rid of for three years. If it didn't sell well on the initial show, they'll rethink it and maybe present it in a different manner to increase sales. That doesn't change the fact that's it's a dud, so you have to stick to the lessons learned here and buy only what's on your list, no matter how enticing they make it sound. ✳

Part II

Fashion

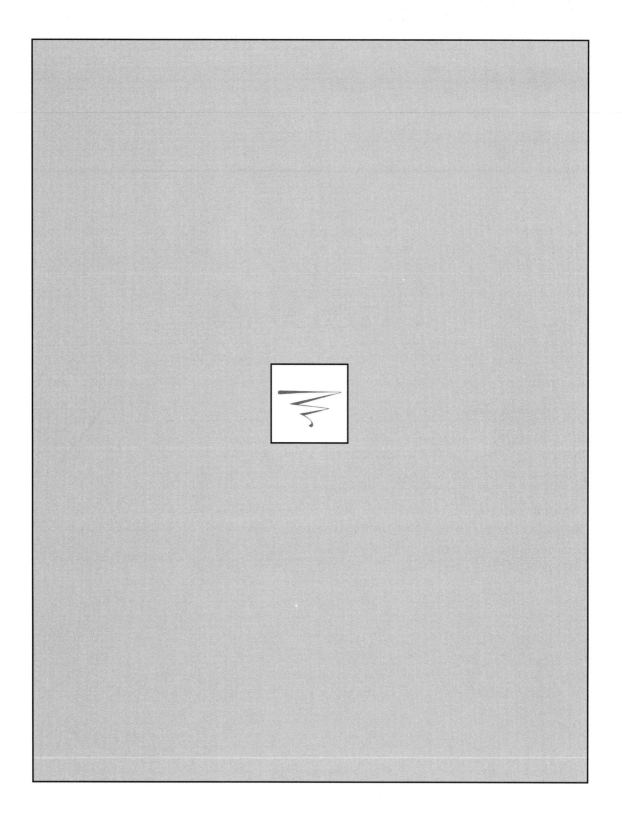

Chapter 5

Stuff You Absolutely
Have to Have

I learned about the basics of a wardrobe out of necessity. My family didn't have much money, and it was important to my mother that her daughter dress well. So not only did I learn to make a lot out of a little, I learned some essential skills that stretched my money and my wardrobe even further.

I believe that you must learn to sew, at least a little bit, either with a needle and thread or with a machine. If you absolutely can't (you can), then you must find a good seamstress to do it for you. Sewing is necessary to take care of the clothes you already own, but also to take advantage of the possibilities of alterations.

When I was younger and poorer, I found a great suit in a very expensive department store. The jacket and skirt were sold separately, and I could afford only one or the other. The sleeves on the jacket were a little long, but I could fix that. Otherwise, it fit perfectly and would work with lots of other skirts I already owned. Still, I really wanted the whole suit. I decided to buy the jacket and then went back to the store every week until the skirt went on sale. Finally it did, but the only skirt left was a size 14. It was too big. If I'd just bought the skirt anyway and "fixed" it by rolling it up or wrapping a big belt around the top, it would have been a mistake. But it wasn't a mistake because I knew how to sew. I took the skirt in, and as a result got a great suit that fit me and my budget.

This is what having the basics in your wardrobe is all about: saving money and looking great. The following are the tools and items of clothing you need in order to build a solid, lasting wardrobe.

Tools

A Sewing Kit/Machine

I learned to sew on an old machine that frequently broke down or veered off in a direction all its own. It was frustrating and took a lot of patience to see a project through. If you learned on a machine like that, I can understand why you think you can't sew. The newer machines—and it doesn't have to be an expensive one—are completely automatic and reliable. The clumsiest person can close a torn seam, make a buttonhole, or even replace a zipper using the special attachments that make it a snap. You can buy a new machine for as little as $150, or pick up a used one for less than $50. After you become adept at using it to fix small problems, you will be inspired to tackle larger ones. It feels so good to salvage a great outfit using your own two hands. You'll see.

If you can't afford a machine—or are just too scared of one—you must have a well-stocked sewing kit. Actually, even if you buy a machine, you should have a sewing kit, too. You won't make repairs if you have to search all over the house for that one needle you know you put somewhere. In your kit have:

* a package of needles in a variety of sizes

* spools of thread (at the very least, black, white, and blue)

* a tin of buttons (put in extra buttons that come with blouses or dresses)

* a seam ripper

* a package of straight pins

Everyone Needs Basics

You would think that since Felicia is dressed by professionals and has access to many, many clothes, that she would not need basics. Not true. Lots of Felicia's outfits utilize the same pieces over and over. She's been wearing the same pair of black suede pumps for seven years. Every time wardrobe tries to throw them out, I dig them out of the trash. Felicia Gallant wears heels every day, but Linda Dano doesn't, so I need shoes that are very, very comfortable since I'm on my feet all day. On days when I can wear those pumps I know I'll be comfortable, and I can concentrate on my acting. So even though they're getting pretty ratty, I still wear them to boost my confidence level. ✳

A Full-length Mirror

As much as you might hate to, you have to look in a mirror to see how you look before you leave the house. Buy a full-length mirror and hang it near your closet, in your bedroom, or in the bathroom—places you know you'll go as you're getting dressed. Also buy a small hand-held mirror so you can see your back.

Ironing Board and Iron

Nothing is worse than wearing a wrinkled outfit that wasn't made to have the "wrinkled look." The best way to avoid wrinkles is to remove clothes from the dryer immediately and hang them in your newly organized closet on the right type of hanger. But if you want to wear something and find it looking crumpled, please iron it first.

You can buy a free-standing ironing board, but if you don't have the space to leave it up all the time, you probably won't use it. If that's the case, try a smaller board that can be installed on a wall or closet door. This type folds down easily for use.

Irons come in all shapes and sizes. A simple steam iron is all you really need. It should have light settings for delicate fabrics and higher ones for stiffer materials. Clean it frequently with a damp sponge and store it near your ironing board.

Dressmaker's Form

This is a luxury item—in terms of cost and space. If you are going to be really serious about the way you dress, it is, however, a must.

Your Own Mannequin

A dressmaker's form is expensive and takes up space that you may not have. I use mine to hem skirts, put together outfits, and to duplicate clothes I already own and love. Of course, you have to be able—or at least willing to learn—to sew.

You can buy a form from a local dressmaker—look in the Yellow Pages—or from one of the following companies. All will ship to you.

Modern Model Form, Inc.
(212) 564–4453
Standard size 8 costs $425. All other sizes and custom forms are more expensive.

Royal Display Form
(212) 575–2679
Sizes 6–16 start at $295. Custom forms are more expensive.

Superior Model Forms Corp.
(212) 947–3633
Sizes 6–16 start at $400. Custom forms are more expensive.

You can also try looking in the classified ads for used forms. If you find one it will probably be a real bargain, under $50. ✹

Clothes
The Suit

Before you decide which pieces to include in your basic wardrobe, you must decide which color your wardrobe is going to be. It has to be black, brown, or navy blue. That doesn't mean you can't wear other colors or even have two wardrobes. I do. I have a black section and a brown section in my closet. I use them separately and mix them together. But to start, pick one color.

You must have a jacket, two skirts, and pair of slacks that are in your basic color and work well together. (If you are buying separates, make sure shades of black, brown, or navy match.) You should buy the best quality you can afford, because you'll be wearing these basics a long time. You really need to know that you have at least one outfit that you can put on anytime and that will make you feel confident and well-dressed.

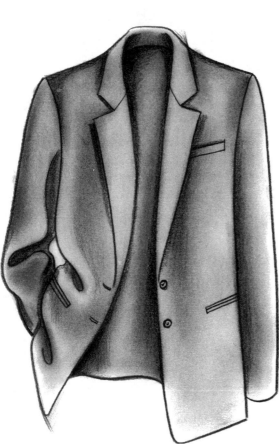

The jacket should be a mid-weight fabric and very plain. Remember, these basics are your blank canvas. We'll paint the picture later. A simple single-breasted style with a plain collar is best.

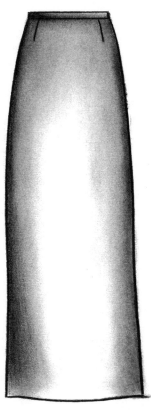
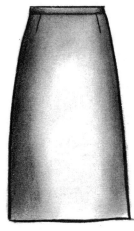

You will need two skirts, one long and one short. The lengths depend on your body type and lifestyle. If you have a lot of evening functions, an ankle-length skirt will get plenty of use, but can still be worn to daytime functions. If your wardrobe is primarily for work, you may choose one above-the-knee length and one just below.

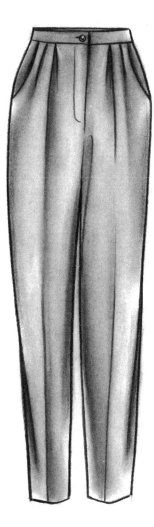

Pants should be comfortable, yet tailored. Choose a fabric that is easy to care for and holds its shape. Lined trousers will last longer. Again, they should be in your basic color and the best quality you can afford.

The Crisp White Blouse

A white cotton blouse is a necessity. Maybe even two. You can wear it with your basic suit, with jeans, even over a swimsuit. The key is to keep it white and crisp. That's where the iron comes into the picture. After washing, iron it to make sure it's ready to go any-time. To keep your shirt bright white, use Rit Color Remover every few months. It's a product developed to remove all color from a garment before re-dying it another color, but it works miracles on whites, too.

The Silky Shirt

Buy one shirt that is a little dressier than your crisp white one, so that you're prepared for more formal occa-sions. This shirt can also be white, or it can be in a brighter color that matches your basic suit. Don't be afraid to buy real silk. The new ones can be washed at home with little fuss.

The Dress

You need one great dress that you can glam up and wear to a cocktail party or tone down for a business meeting. This isn't a one-time-only special-occasion dress, but one that you can wear over and over again. It has to be in your basic color so you can wear it with your basic jacket. If you have nice arms, this dress should be short-sleeved to carry you through every season. If you'd rather cover your arms, then this dress should be in a lightweight fabric, again to be appropriate for all seasons. It should have a simple style—maybe an A-line or sheath—with few details.

Shop for this dress when you don't need it. If you're rushed to find something for your friend's wedding *this* Saturday, you won't take the time to make sure the dress meets all of your needs and you'll be stuck with yet another one-occasion dress.

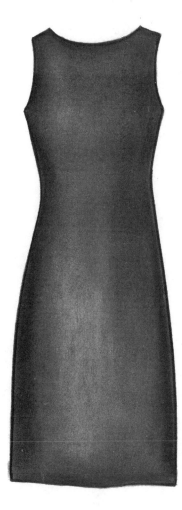

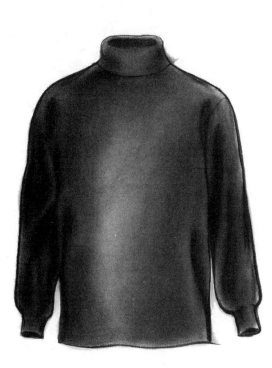

The Sweater

You probably own many turtlenecks or other simple, soft sweaters, but you need to make sure you have one in your basic color. You may also need a white one. You can wear this light sweater under your crisp white shirt for a layered look, or you may wear it alone with your jacket and skirt.

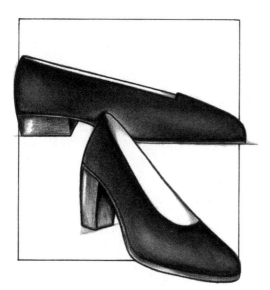

The Shoes

If your basic color is black, buy black basic shoes. If it's navy, buy navy. You need one pair of flat shoes in your basic color and one pair of medium-heel (one and a half inches) pumps. They should be sturdy and the best quality you can afford. Leather-soled shoes should be taken immediately to the shoemaker and resoled in rubber to last longer.

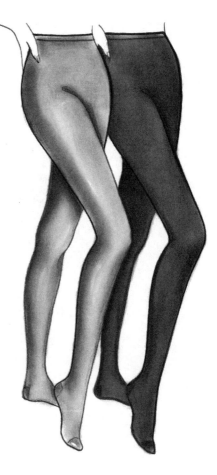

The Hose/The Socks

Buy a few pair of hose and socks in your basic color. Navy wearers: Buy navy. Not light blue, not blue/black, but true navy. Bring your skirt to the store to match the color if you have to. I think you need at least one pair of opaque for day and one pair of sheer hose for evening.

The Winter Coat

You will need one good coat, preferably mid-calf length.
You can buy it in your basic color or in a color that goes
with the basics. If your wardrobe is brown, a red coat will
look terrific. But remember, once you commit to another
color you must then buy only accessories that go with
that color *and* your basic color. You are now married to
that color. When you buy a scarf, it has to be both red and
brown to tie everything together.

The Handbag

Buy one good handbag in your basic color. You can wear
black with navy, but for now try to stick with a one-color
plan until you get really good at this. Buy a medium-size bag
that fits the stuff you need to carry around. A too-big bag
will weigh you, and your outfit, down. One too small will
look overstuffed and messy.

Buy a wallet. Now, of course, this can be any color
you like, but it has to be big
enough to hold everything
neatly. There's no point in
my getting you all organized
if you are going to just
shove money and dry-
cleaner receipts into your
bag or pockets. You have to
look pulled together from
head to toe.

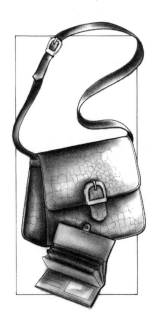

The Belt

Buy a belt in your basic black, brown, or navy-blue color, but pay attention to the buckle. If the buckle is metal, you have to decide whether you are going to wear gold tones or silver tones. If you wear silver jewelry one day and gold the next, you may need to buy two belts, each with a different color buckle.

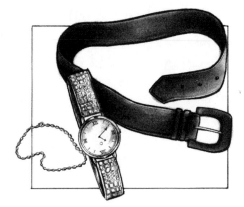

The Watch

Most of us wear a watch, but some pay little attention to whether or not it matches our outfits. I use watches as accessories, so I have many. But to start, you need one that can go from day to evening and not be noticed. To keep it simple, choose a gold- or silver-toned watch with few details. If you buy a brightly colored watch you will need to wear those colors every day you wear the watch, and that's no fun.

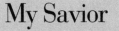

My Savior

Basics are not clothes that just hang in your closet, which you wear every now and then. Basics are the pieces that you wear constantly; these are the clothes that make you feel comfortable and confident. You have to love them and know that you look great when you start your outfit with them. I have a pair—actually I'm now on my second pair—of black gabardine slacks that I wear at least twice a week. Gabardine is a durable fabric that hangs beautifully and packs easily without wrinkling. These pants are like a safety net for me. They fit when I'm five pounds on the heavy side or when I'm feeling bloated. Since I can never eat without dropping something on myself, I don't have to worry when I'm wearing these slacks; they hide everything. I love them so much, I recently bought an off-white pair for the summer. ✻

In future chapters, I'll show you how you can take these few items and add to them to create a business/daytime wardrobe, an evening wardrobe, and a leisure/travel wardrobe. But really, this is all the stuff that you truly need. These are the basics. If you had only the items on the above list, you could dress well forever. Of course, it wouldn't be as much fun as learning to shop and pulling together other outfits, but if you had to, you could get by with just the basics.

Basic Checklist

Tools

* Sewing Machine/Kit
* Full-length Mirror
* Ironing Board and Iron
* Dressmaker's Form

Clothes

* Suit
  * Jacket
  * Two Skirts (long and short)
  * Slacks
* Crisp White Blouse
* Silky Shirt
* All-purpose Dress
* Sweater
* Shoes (flats and pumps)
* Hose/Socks
* Coat
* Handbag
* Belt
* Watch

Fashion Victim to Fashion Plate

Talk-show host Leeza Gibbons remembers a time when she would adapt whatever style was out there, not caring that "I looked totally stupid. I thought being fashionable was dressing just like the magazines said I should. Or copying what the biggest stars were doing. It took a long time for me to realize that trying to be someone else wasn't going to work for me."

Leeza used to follow every trend. When the Farrah Fawcett hairdo was in, Leeza was the first in line. Dark, smoky, Angie Dickinson eyes? Leeza had 'em. But other women's signature looks didn't translate into real style for her. She had to find her own way. And she has.

"My style now is a sleeker, more classic look. I still have tons of black, but I also use brown as a basic color, mixed with creams and camels. I wear purple as my bright color."

By sticking to her basics, which complement her classic looks, I think Leeza now dresses beautifully. Others do, too. She was included in *People* magazine's 10 Best-Dressed List in 1996. She really deserves the honor. ✳

Chapter 6

Putting It All Together—for Work

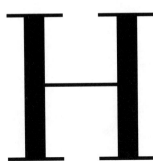ere's where you'll begin to make the move from just having clothes to having a wardrobe that shows your style. You could wear your basics every day and probably get away with it, but then you would just be wearing a uniform. Black suit, white shirt, black pumps. That would be okay, but it's not style. What is style? You may recognize bad style when you see it—a baggy red jacket with a wrinkled blouse underneath, loose buttons, a too-tight dress. Great style is quieter. One of the most visible clues to great style is simplicity. You may not pick a really stylish woman out of a crowd because her clothes—her frame—are so simple. I don't mean boring, or safe. It's something different.

Go to Saks or Bergdorf's or whatever high-end store is in your area and look at the women who shop there. They look pulled together. Their suits are pressed, their shoes are polished, they are not wearing head-to-toe blinding "look at me" clothes. These are real women who need clothes that work every day. You can't look at celebrities to find this kind of style because celebrities *do* wear clothes that make people notice them or that complement their stage personalities.

Most designers' "real" styles—the ones that make it to the stores, not just shown on the runway—are subdued (unless their claim to fame is flash, like Pucci in the sixties or Versace now). They use solid colors like black, navy, gray, or soft brown for the main pieces in their collections, the classic pieces stores always have in stock. If they add color it will be to blouses, vests, or scarves—not jackets and skirts. Now, I know this does not match up with the images you see in magazines and on TV, but you have to remember that many of those images are of models or celebrities, not the kind of woman like you who works every day in an office. Style isn't about showing your money, either. Even very wealthy women dress simply during the day. Their style is in the details and accessories, just like yours should be.

Our job now is to take your basics and other clothes you already have and add the pieces that will give you a selection of outfits that look great every day.

Clothes Speak Volumes

How you dress at work reflects not only who you are, but what you're capable of. My theory is that you should always dress for the job you want next, not the one you have now. So what if you're in an entry-level position? It's up to you to transmit the image of someone far more accomplished than your job title implies. It's called Dressing for Success. Okay, that's a cliché. But it's a cliché that works. When you present a pulled-together, detailed appearance, people (your bosses) believe that your work habits are organized and thorough, too.

Upwardly mobile dressing is only one part of your office attitude. You also have to consider what type of business you're in and observe how other, successful employees dress. If you're in banking, accounting, or law, it's fine to wear tailored, quiet suits. But just because you work on Wall Street, you shouldn't feel like you have to dress like a man. You can still look feminine *and* businesslike. If you're in a more creative field, like graphic design or publishing, you'll look stodgy and out of place in such formal clothes.

Showing Too Much

Needing to save money for college, I once worked in a factory. Yes, a factory! On the assembly line even. I felt very grown-up and tried to dress up for my new role every day. I thought things were going really swell until the day the floor manager called me into his office. Apparently, I had been attracting too much attention from the other, mostly male, workers. My work was fine, but my clothes were too fitted and revealing. It was true. I looked around and noticed that I was wrong. Yes, my clothes were revealing, but they were also too dressy for this type of work. I was showing my coworkers up. You really have to pay attention to what the people who work around you are wearing. You want to be stylish, but you want to fit in, too. ✳

Where to Start

Office dressing is all about separates. Each piece you buy must go well with all the items you already own. You should be able to pop out of bed, hit the shower, then select a great outfit within minutes. If you stand in front of your closet every morning debating over this or that, you haven't done your homework. I have no idea what is in your closet except for the basics, which I know you've assembled by now. On the following pages, I am going to suggest the styles and pieces I think you need to make dressing for work easy, every single day.

Dressing for Success

I once had a woman come to Strictly Personal (I have run this personal shopping business for more than ten years) for help because she felt the way she was dressing for work wasn't getting her anywhere. As soon as I saw her wardrobe, I diagnosed the problem in two seconds. She was choosing the styles and shapes that looked good on her and were professional. The problem was in the fabrics. She was skimping on quality so she could afford more clothes. I had her start from scratch and assemble the basics in good, quality fabrics. Along the way she learned how to tell the difference. Now she had less to wear, but she makes a bigger impact. Within months she had moved into a more demanding position, and I'm sure the change in her wardrobe was a major cause of it. ✳

10 Easy Pieces

All you need to dress well for work are your basics and ten other separates. Before you begin assembling your work wardrobe, you need to decide what your third and fourth colors are going to be. Black, brown, or navy is your first color, white is your second, so you need to add two more. Having more than four colors makes your wardrobe just a bunch of clothes and makes it harder to dress easily. Choose a soft third color, such as tan, camel, gray, French blue, yellow, etc., and a bright fourth color, such as red, purple, teal, etc. Once you've made your choice, you can't buy anything that's not in one (or more) of those four colors.

Add these ten separates for a complete work wardrobe:

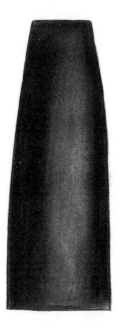

1. LONG SKIRT IN BLACK, BROWN, OR NAVY (YOUR BASIC COLOR)

This should be a straight-cut skirt falling just above ankle length. The beauty of this purchase is that it is serious enough for work, but elegant enough (with a change of accessories) for evening.

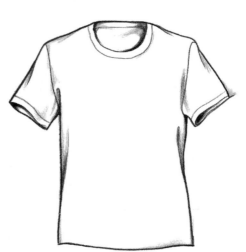

2. WHITE COTTON T-SHIRTS

Plain round-neck Hanes T-shirts (sold in three-packs) are terrific. Iron before wear for a crisp look. Tip: If you are large and shirt is snug around hips, cut sides and stitch flaps to finish.

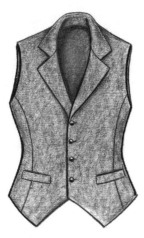

3. VEST IN YOUR BASIC COLOR

Fabric should have some texture, but no other colors. You can wear this instead of a jacket. If arms are firm, wear with a white T-shirt underneath.

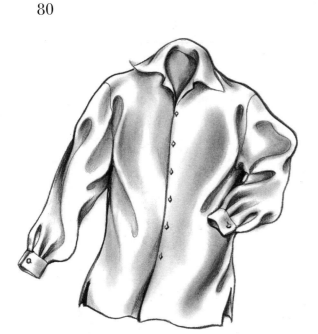

4. SOFTER FABRIC BLOUSE (COTTON, RAYON, ETC.)

This should be in your "bright" color. I would choose red or a mustardy yellow for a black wardrobe; French blue or a purple for a brown wardrobe; and red for a navy wardrobe. You can choose a print if you want, as long as it only contains your four colors and no others.

5. SILK BLOUSE

Tailored enough to wear to work, silk to carry over into evening. This should be in your "soft" color. I use tan as my soft color for my black and brown wardrobe. You might use gray or yellow for a navy wardrobe.

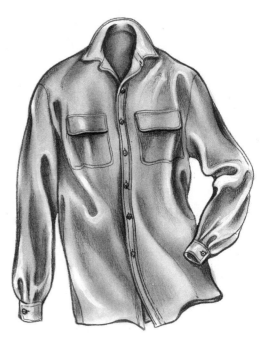

6. UNCONSTRUCTED JACKET

This should be in your soft color. You can wear it with your skirt or, on casual days, with your slacks; with your white T-shirt or cotton blouse. Wear with jeans on days off.

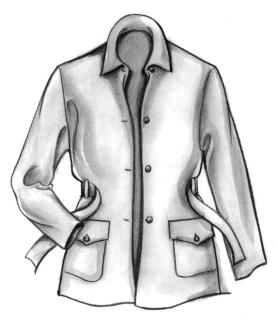

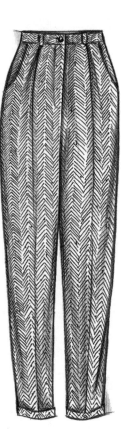

7. PRINT SLACKS

Find a tweed or small plaid that has two or more of your colors in weave; a black, tan, and white tweed would be perfect for a black wardrobe; a tan, brown, and white tweed for a brown wardrobe; navy, gray, and white for a navy wardrobe. If you don't wear slacks to work often, choose a tweed skirt instead.

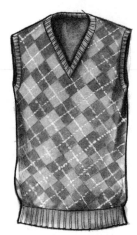

8. COLORED VEST

Find an interesting textured fabric in either your soft or bright color. I chose red to wear with my black suit, my tweed slacks and black jacket, and with my long skirt and silk blouse.

9. CARDIGAN SWEATER

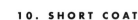

You can wear this in place of a jacket. It can have buttons or be unconstructed with no buttons. If you can find a sweater set (comes with a matching short-sleeved sweater to wear underneath), buy it. I chose black, but you could choose a cardigan in either your basic color or your soft or bright colors.

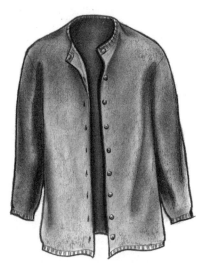

10. SHORT COAT

A short coat is really just a bigger, longer, heavier jacket. This one should be about thigh length. Some people call them car coats or pea coats. You can wear slacks and a blouse, throw on your coat, and go. A safe choice is one in your basic color, but you can also choose a coat in your bright or soft color.

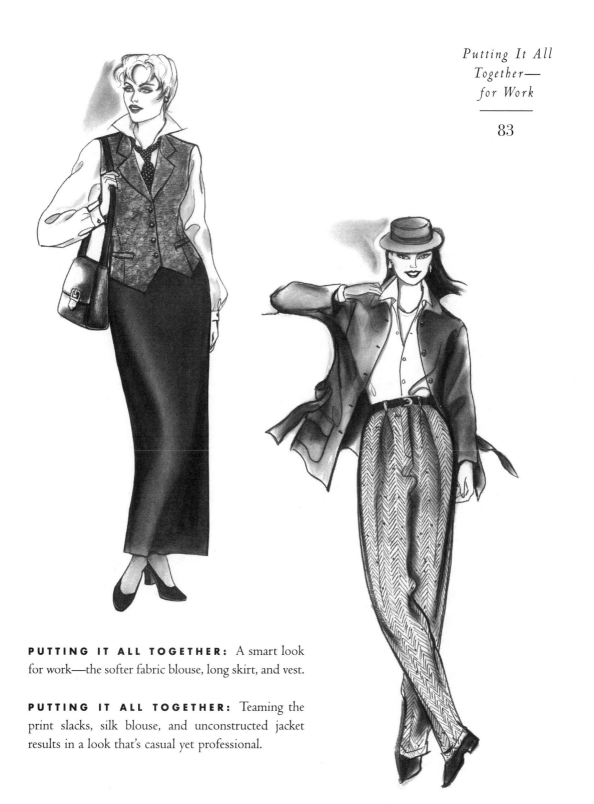

PUTTING IT ALL TOGETHER: A smart look for work—the softer fabric blouse, long skirt, and vest.

PUTTING IT ALL TOGETHER: Teaming the print slacks, silk blouse, and unconstructed jacket results in a look that's casual yet professional.

Fabrics That Work

Your basics and your work wardrobe should be made from durable, seasonless fabrics.

Gabardine

This is a closely woven fabric with definite ridges caused by the warp-faced twill weave. This fabric is made in either cotton, wool, or rayon. Good gabardine is expensive, but it will pay for itself over the years. It retains its shape, is fairly wrinkle-free, and wears well year-round. A good choice for basic suit, skirts, and especially slacks.

Crepe

This fabric is matte (not shiny), very finely wrinkled and has a textured finish. Crepe can be made from wool, cotton, or silk, or from a blend. Crepe washes and wears well year-round. A good choice for blouses and skirts.

Jersey

A tightly woven, lightweight fabric made from wool, rayon, or man-made fibers. Can often be machine-washed and, if removed promptly from dryer, wrinkle-free. Wears year-round. A good choice for blouses and skirts.

Tweed

A coarse wool fabric woven with a mix of colors. Tweed holds shape well, but usually must be dry-cleaned. A lightweight tweed can be worn year-round. Best for jackets, vests, and slacks.

Fibers are what fabrics are made from. Natural fibers, such as cotton, linen, wool, and silk feel better to wear, but wrinkle more easily than synthetics and may not last as long.

Cotton

A vegetable fiber, cotton is comfortable year-round. It is often mixed with a synthetic fiber to reduce wrinkling and increase wear. Best for basic crisp white shirt, T-shirts, and undergarments.

Wool

An animal fiber, wool is made from different animal fleeces to create different fabrics such as cashmere, camel hair, mohair, angora. Fleece from lambs is used for most standard wool garments. Wool is also often mixed with other fibers, such as cotton. Good wool is wrinkle-resistant, wears well, and will hold shape if properly cared for. Best for basic suits, skirts, slacks, coats.

Silk

Silk is cultivated from silkworms and is a very fine yet strong fiber. Raw silk is created when the worm's natural gum is not cleaned from the fiber. Pure silk requires gentle care and is not recommended for everyday wear. Silk blends wear better and work best for blouses. Washable silk is just that, silk garments that can be machine-washed.

Double Work

I have an unusual job because I go to work and then get dressed. Actors don't have to look perfect when they walk in the door because they have hair and makeup and wardrobe people at their beck and call. I, however, come to work fully dressed every day. My coworkers tease me to no end about it, but I can't seem to leave the house without looking totally pulled together. I arrived looking so good when I was working on *As the World Turns,* that the wardrobe department eventually just asked me to dress myself. The whole time I was on that show I was my own dresser. ✳

Synthetic Fibers

Used to be synthetic meant scratchy, shiny polyester. Advances in fiber technology have led to better, more wearable fibers that provide good wear and ease of care. A blend of natural and synthetic fibers takes the best qualities of each to create natural-feeling fabrics that are also durable.

Nylon

First used to make hosiery, it is now often mixed with crepes and twills for blouses.

Polyester

Polyester alone can still feel uncomfortable and hot, but when mixed with cotton or wool it strengthens fabric for durability and longer wear. Used to make all types of clothing.

Rayon

Also called viscose, good rayon can look and feel like silk. When mixed with cotton or silk it adds durability and washability to garments. Mixed with wool for suits, skirts, and slacks.

Now You Have to Dress Down?

The fact is, the world is slowly becoming more casual. In the past five years, just about every company has instituted casual Fridays or other selected days when employees can dress down. Some companies even let employees buy extra casual days by donating to chosen charities. You, who have worked hard to put together a professional look, are now faced with the option of choosing casual, comfortable clothes to wear on dress-down days. What to do?

The first, and most obvious, thing to do is to look around and see what everyone else is wearing, especially your boss. While it's important to look professional, even on casual days, you don't want to be the only one wearing a formal suit. You'll stand out and will be marked as someone who is not a team player.

If you usually wear a suit or a jacket and skirt to work, you can wear your basic slacks and crisp white shirt on casual days. You should still bring a jacket, even if you don't wear it all day, just in case an important meeting comes up unexpectedly. Don't make the mistake of going too casual. If your boss is wearing jeans, you can, too. But don't wear torn jeans, unpressed shirts, or a skirt without pantyhose. Strappy sandals and clothes that are revealing are best left at home, too.

Work Wardrobe Checklist

✳ Ankle-length skirt in basic color

✳ White cotton T-shirts

✳ Vest in basic color

✳ Softer fabric blouse in bright color

✳ Silk blouse in soft color

✳ Unconstructed jacket in soft color

✳ Print slacks

✳ Colored vest in bright or soft color, or print

✳ Cardigan sweater in basic, bright, or soft color

✳ Short coat in basic, bright, or soft color

Chapter 7

Putting It All Together—for Evening

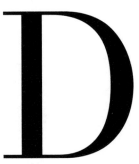

Dressing for cocktail parties, weddings, benefits, or a night at the theater doesn't necessarily mean assembling a completely separate wardrobe, which you wear only at night. Truly stylish women—which you're now becoming—learn to be creative and use their daytime wardrobe (and basics) as a base for evening wear. Of course, there will always be those special occasions for which you'll want to buy a stunning new dress or suit, and you should, as long as it fits into your overall wardrobe plan and you can afford it.

It used to be that rules for dressing for an evening out were pretty cut-and-dried. If you went to the theater, you wore your very best. For a wedding, you knew that black and white were definitely out. If an invitation read "black-tie," a floor-length dress was the only option. These days those rules do not hold as true. Women wear a range of styles, from blue jeans to sequined finery, to attend an opera (not that I think that's okay). Wedding guests wear whatever they want, and black-tie covers a range of styles. Without instructions it's hard for women to know just what to wear. That's why I believe in trying to keep it simple.

Start with the Basics

Evening is the reason I told you to include a simple black, or navy, or brown dress in your basic wardrobe. Ideally this dress should be made from a fabric you can wear year-round, such as jersey, crepe, or raw silk. The best style is a simple, straight, short-sleeved sheath that falls an inch or two above your knee, depending on your height. It shouldn't be so slinky and sexy that you can't also wear this dress to work under a tailored jacket. It may take you months to find this dress. You should shop for it now, before you really need it. Take the time to find the dress that fits you perfectly. You have to feel absolutely comfortable every time you put it on. If you are constantly pulling, tugging, or struggling to breathe when you wear this dress, you will never want to wear it. Earmark a big chunk of your budget for this purchase, because you want to find "the" dress and not be held back by cost when you do find it. Don't hesitate to have the dress tailored or shortened if it is almost "the" dress, but needs some fine-tuning.

So you have the perfect basic dress and I know you also have simple pumps in your basic color (if not, go buy them and then read the rest of this chapter). You could wear these two items—with matching hose—and go just about anywhere without looking out of place. You may not stand out from the crowd, but no one is going to say, "Who is the woman in that awful chartreuse pantsuit?" either. You won't look stylish, but you can get away with it because you will look neat and organized. But, and here's the good news, you can add to your basic attire and turn it into stunning evening wear.

Magic Tricks

I attend many dressy functions: awards shows, benefits, things like that. I also work full-time on *Another World*, design and sell accessories on QVC, run Strictly Personal, and occasionally I'll fit in a movie or other acting project. I am busy, busy, busy. I get an invitation for yet another night out, and I don't have time to go shopping, nor do I really want to add to my wardrobe more clothes that I know I won't wear that often. Yet I have to wear something, and I have to look good because I am in the public eye. I'll hear about it or see some awful picture in a magazine if I don't look fashionable. So for those evenings, I turn to my button collection as my savior. My best fashion trick is to take a simple black jacket (probably one I've had copied) and change the simple buttons to fancy, sparkling ones. It takes ten minutes to sew on new buttons and I up the glamour quotient 100 percent. I pull on a long skirt, and—voilà!—I'm ready for evening. ✳

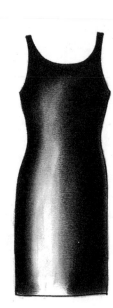

10 Easy Pieces

1. COCKTAIL DRESS
IN BLACK, BROWN, OR NAVY

A little sexier than your basic dress. Add accessories, jacket, hose, and you can go anywhere.

2. LONG SKIRT
IN BLACK, BROWN, OR NAVY

This is also part of your work wardrobe. With a change of accessories it becomes evening.

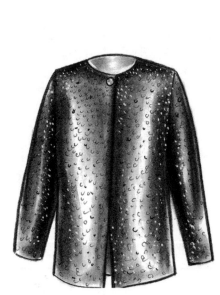

3. GLITTERY JACKET

It's the fabric that makes this jacket evening wear (never wear it during the day). Silver, gold, or colored sequins (in your bright color) are great.

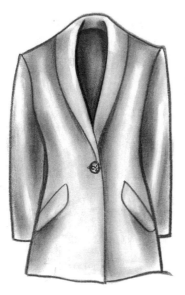

4. WHITE HEAVY SILK JACKET

You can wear this over your cocktail dress, with a long skirt or chiffon pants.

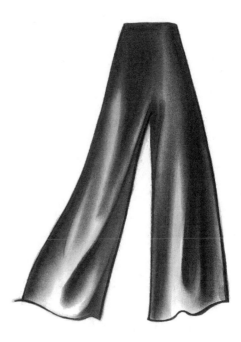

5. SILK OR CHIFFON PANTS IN BASIC, BRIGHT, OR SOFT COLOR

Soft, loose palazzo pants under a jacket are dressy enough for any occasion.

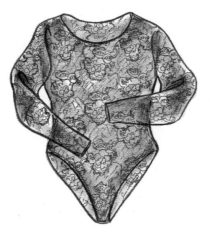

6. LACE OR GLITTERY BODYSUIT

Choose black or white for versatility. You may be able to wear it without a bra under a jacket (many have built-in support). A bodysuit is not for those without a defined waist; choose a loose-fitting lace over-blouse instead.

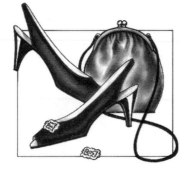

7. SUEDE PUMPS IN BASIC COLOR

Choose an open-toe or higher heel than you would wear for day.

8. EVENING BAG IN BASIC COLOR

Choose a bag without gold or silver trim to avoid clashing with jewelry.

9. SHAWL IN BASIC OR BRIGHT COLOR

On cooler evenings it can work as your coat. A shawl can dress up any outfit.

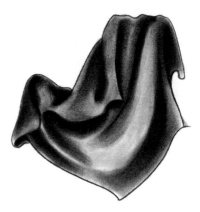

Pumping Up Pumps

Plain black pumps—or navy or brown—can be easily turned into evening shoes with the addition of shoe clips. Shoe clips were more popular in the fifties and you can find many rhinestone styles in antique stores or flea markets (a good investment, they can also be worn as jewelry clipped onto jacket pockets). Modern versions are available in accessory departments or those stores that sell only accessories. ✳

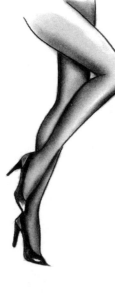

10. SHEER HOSE

Evening calls for smooth, sexy legs. Save opaque hose for day.

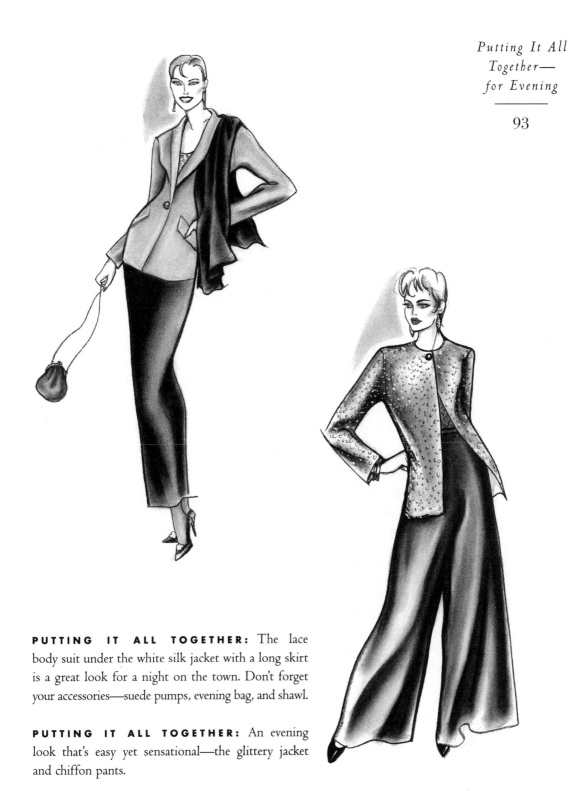

PUTTING IT ALL TOGETHER: The lace body suit under the white silk jacket with a long skirt is a great look for a night on the town. Don't forget your accessories—suede pumps, evening bag, and shawl.

PUTTING IT ALL TOGETHER: An evening look that's easy yet sensational—the glittery jacket and chiffon pants.

Evening Fabrics
Chiffon

A sheer fabric that falls loosely. Made from silk or synthetics. Great for skirts and slacks.

Faille

A lightweight fabric made from silk or synthetics. Great for skirts and slacks.

Gabardine

When made from silk, it is lightweight yet holds shape. Better-grade silk gabardine is great for jackets and slacks.

Georgette

Sheer, lightweight, and wrinkle-proof. Made from silk or synthetics. Great for skirts and slacks and dresses (must be lined).

Lamé

A lightweight fabric woven with metallic threads. Made from silk, cotton, wool, or synthetics. Best for jackets, blouses, or sweaters.

Satin

A shiny, lustrous fabric made from silk, synthetics, or a blend. Great for shawls, evening jackets, or slacks.

Where Are You Going?

I have a friend who has a rack full of sequined blouses and shimmery dresses. She keeps buying these things because as soon as she enters a store she is attracted to the flash. The problem is she never goes anyplace where these clothes are appropriate. She doesn't have a huge social life and rarely attends events that require such fancy dressing (she doesn't even like to go out!). You shouldn't make this mistake: spend a lot of your wardrobe budget on clothes that are inappropriate for your lifestyle. Think about what you do, where you go, and how other women dress at those events. If you go out to a dressy event twice a year, don't stock up on evening clothes, even if you love them. ✳

Evening Wardrobe Checklist

✹ Cocktail dress

✹ Long skirt (from your work wardrobe)

✹ Glittery jacket

✹ White heavy silk jacket

✹ Silk or chiffon loose pants

✹ Lace or glittery bodysuit

✹ Suede pumps

✹ Shawl

✹ Sheer hose

✹ Evening bag

It Pays to Rent

Y ou don't have to spend $1,000 on an evening gown to attend that once-a-year black-tie event. Many cities, even smaller ones, now have stores that rent formal attire (look in the Yellow Pages under FORMAL WEAR) for very reasonable prices. You may pay $200 for one night's use, but you get a brand-new dress that no one's ever seen you in before and you don't have to dry-clean (the store will do it) or store it in your closet. (Renting makes real sense if you're pregnant. I mean, when will you ever wear *that* dress again!) Many stores will often alter the dress to fit, too. The best part is that next year you get to rent another brand-new dress! ✹

Chapter 8

Putting It All
Together—for Leisure

It's really tempting to wake up on a Saturday morning and throw on a pair of raggy sweatpants (unless you paid attention in Chapter 3 and tossed them) and an old T-shirt, isn't it? It's your day off, you have to do the laundry, vacuum, wash the kitchen floor, so why not dress comfortably? You *can* wear raggy clothes around the house. It makes sense to pull on comfy standbys sometimes, but you can still look pulled together and be comfortable. It's a matter of assembling a leisure wardrobe that works for you on your time off, when you're most likely to slip into your old Sweatshopper or Size-Impaired ways.

So what do you do for fun? Do you spend weekends at flea markets and antique stores like I do? Do you run errands on Saturday, go to church on Sunday? Go to the movies, host dinner parties, play golf? If you're a stay-at-home mom, most of your wardrobe will fall into this category, so pay attention. First, make a list—yes, another one—of the type of leisure activities you participate in the most. We have to find out where you go and who's going to see you there. You may not care who you run into at the supermarket, but it may be a different story at the PTA meeting. I *am* trying to teach you to dress well for yourself, but let's face it, we all care about what other people think of us and do sort of dress for them, too. If you assemble a never-fail leisure wardrobe, you can be ready in minutes to face whatever comes up.

Here's what my typical weekend looks like, and what I wear when I'm not working:

Frank and I usually head for our house in Connecticut on the weekends. There we spend a lot of time gardening, driving into town in our vintage Ford truck, visiting with friends, and basically just poking around. Just like you, I have to do food shopping and house cleaning, as well as other weekend chores. For most of these activities I have a weekend uniform: white Hanes T-shirt or turtleneck, white sweatpants, white socks, white sneakers, and if it's chilly, a white cotton vest. Okay, so I look like Mr. Clean. (I have the exact same outfit in black, too). But it works for me. I'm comfortable, yet look pulled together. I can wear this outfit into town, but I can also quickly change to my basic slacks and pumps, toss on my basic jacket, and be ready to go anywhere in minutes.

If we are going out to dinner or having friends in, I generally wear the same type of clothes I would in New York; that means maybe adding a nicer blouse to my basic slacks and jacket. I would probably also add some earrings, a necklace, and a belt. See how simple it can be?

You may have noticed that I start with my basics and build from there. Your basics are always there for you; that's why they're so important. The three basic pieces you'll rely on over and over again in putting together your leisure wardrobe are your crisp white shirt, your flat shoes, and the jacket from your basic suit. These items, a few soft cotton shirts, and a pair of jeans or casual slacks may be all you need to get through a typical day off. I have a friend who wears the same Harvé Bernard navy jacket and Gucci loafers just about every day. She pairs them with a simple white shirt and pressed jeans, yet

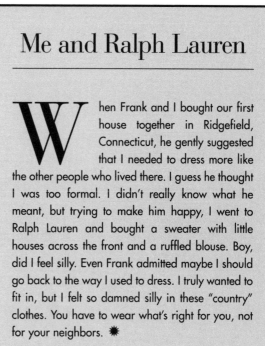

Me and Ralph Lauren

When Frank and I bought our first house together in Ridgefield, Connecticut, he gently suggested that I needed to dress more like the other people who lived there. I guess he thought I was too formal. I didn't really know what he meant, but trying to make him happy, I went to Ralph Lauren and bought a sweater with little houses across the front and a ruffled blouse. Boy, did I feel silly. Even Frank admitted maybe I should go back to the way I used to dress. I truly wanted to fit in, but I felt so damned silly in these "country" clothes. You have to wear what's right for you, not for your neighbors. ✳

looks tailored and well-dressed all the time. Of course, she adds a different scarf or pin each time for a little individuality, but really she is wearing her "uniform" every day. It may sound a little boring, and I kid her to death about wearing the same thing, but even I have to admit she looks good in those clothes. She knows it and it shows. She feels confident knowing that her appearance is taken care of. Now, I'm not suggesting you do the same thing. What I want you to do is assemble a few of these uniforms that you can call on when you need them. My friend certainly wouldn't wear this outfit when she takes her kids to the playground, but she does have another ready-to-go look that works for that situation.

10 Easy Pieces

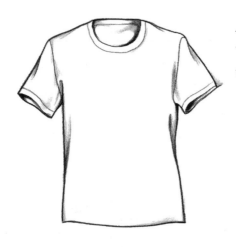

1. WHITE COTTON T-SHIRTS

You can live in these. Wear them alone or under a vest or jacket.

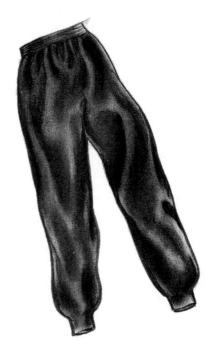

White Makes Sense

Y ou may wonder why I suggest wearing all white for leisure. You're thinking, *It gets so dirty and stains easily.* The reason I prefer whites is that you can bleach them. You'll get the same stains as you would on blue or green or pink, but they're easier to remove from whites. I have a fifteen-year-old white gabardine coat that I was minutes away from throwing out when I decided to bleach it. I'd put off using bleach because I was worried about damaging the fabric, but it was so stained I was going to get rid of it anyway, so why not? I learned that if you are gentle, you can bleach just about anything. I filled the washer, added a cup of bleach, and just let it soak. I then ran it through clean water, and believe it or not, all of the stains came out (I scrubbed the cuffs with a toothbrush to remove tough stains). ✳

2. BLACK/WHITE SWEATPANTS

Buy good-quality 100 percent cotton, or a cotton/polyester blend. Get a good fit: not too tight, not too baggy. Holes or stains are not allowed.

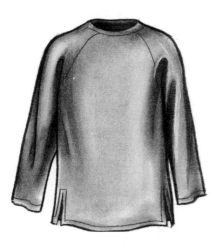

3. SWEATSHIRTS

Buy black and white, but also other bright colors you like.

4. BLACK OR WHITE CARDIGAN SWEATER

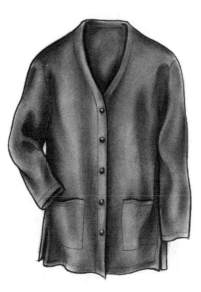

Buy cotton or cotton blend. Can double as casual jacket.

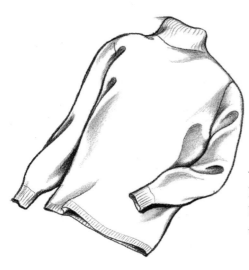

5. BLACK AND WHITE TURTLENECKS

For colder days. Buy cotton or cotton blend. You can wear these alone or under jacket or vest.

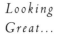

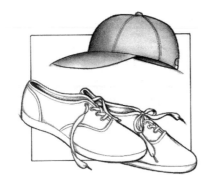

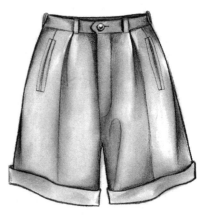

6. WHITE SNEAKERS

As little detail as possible. I have a pair of slip-ons and a pair that lace. The slip-ons are a little (just a little) more formal.

7. BASEBALL CAPS

Saturday morning is a notorious bad hair day. A cap makes you look stylish.

8. BLACK, WHITE, KHAKI SHORTS

I don't wear shorts often—okay, never—but I'm not you. Use same fit guidelines you would for slacks.

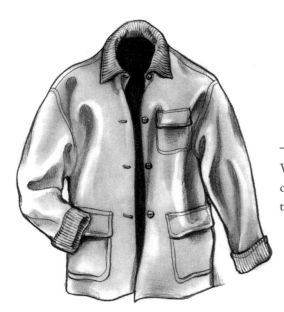

9. SHORT JACKET

White or basic color. Buy cotton
or gabardine. Lightweight, about
thigh length.

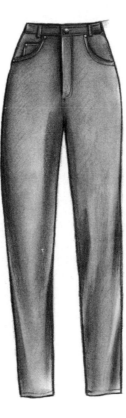

10. JEANS

I never wear them, but realize most people live
in them. Just make sure they fit, are clean and
not torn.

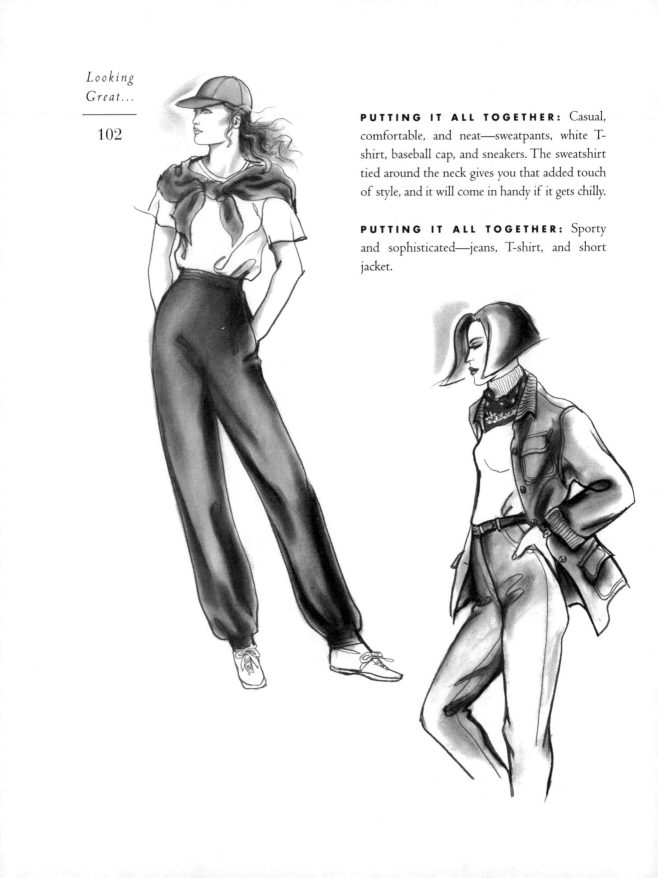

PUTTING IT ALL TOGETHER: Casual, comfortable, and neat—sweatpants, white T-shirt, baseball cap, and sneakers. The sweatshirt tied around the neck gives you that added touch of style, and it will come in handy if it gets chilly.

PUTTING IT ALL TOGETHER: Sporty and sophisticated—jeans, T-shirt, and short jacket.

That Dirty Little Word

I can take just about anything, but say the word "swimsuit" and I start to shake. Say "bikini" and I just about faint. If you're like me, shopping for (and wearing) a swimsuit makes you break out in hives. But, of course, you have to have one. Everyone likes to go to the beach or pool every now and then. There aren't signs that say "No Fatties Allowed." We all have the right to relax and enjoy a good dip; it's the finding something to wear part that scares us away.

Good fit and flattering styles are the key to feeling confident while wearing a swimsuit. Unfortunately, the only way to be really sure what works is to try on, and try on, piles of suits. You don't have to go in blind, though. Here are some fit tips for all types of bodies:

Full Hips and Thighs

AVOID: Tight leg openings, horizontal stripes, belted suits, very high-cut or boy-cut (too low) legs.

LOOK FOR: Lighter shades on top, neckline details, wide-set shoulder straps. They all draw the eye up and away from hips and thighs. A full cut in the back and high leg openings flatter this type of figure.

No Waist

AVOID: Single color with side seams, horizontal seams, or other horizontal details at waist, high-waisted bikinis.

LOOK FOR: Suits with curving side panels (often in another color). Also, busy patterns that don't let the eye focus on one spot. Hip-hugger bikinis.

Small Bust

AVOID: Plain athletic tanks, anything strapless or with a high neckline.

LOOK FOR: Suits with detail along bustline. Ruffles, appliqués, shirring add depth. Built-in push-up bras do the job for you. Wear bright colors on top.

Large Bust

AVOID: Lightweight fabrics, strapless or high-necked tops. Too thin straps and low backs offer little support.

LOOK FOR: Support bras sewn in, heavier fabrics, wide straps, solid colors on top (breasts stretch prints out of shape).

Long Torso

AVOID: Anything too short (J. Crew, Land's End, Eddie Bauer catalogs now sell suits by torso measurements). Vertical stripes, low-cut bikinis, high necks, or boy-cut legs.

LOOK FOR: Bikinis, belts, horizontal stripes, waist details, and high-cut legs all cut length of torso.

On the Road

I travel a lot for work and am often in airports. One trend that really bothers me is the way people now dress for plane travel. Most women look like they are dressed to sit on the couch with the remote control, eating potato chips. The person who invented hot-pink leggings (and then made them in size 3X) should be shot. I can't stand this! You should dress to travel. I don't mean wear a business suit and pantyhose, but wear something that makes you look attractive. You're still out in public when you're on a plane; it isn't your living room, dress a little. Your basic slacks, a white T-shirt, and basic jacket are (or should be) plenty comfortable to wear on a plane. ✳

Over the Suit

Once again, pull out your crisp white shirt. It makes the perfect swimsuit cover-up. You can also buy a sheerer version that you only wear to the beach. Not only will it cover your suit, it will offer some protection from the sun. Also buy a short wrap skirt or a sarong or pareo.

Leisure Wardrobe Checklist

* White T-shirts
* Black and white sweatpants
* Sweatshirts
* Cardigan sweater, black or white cotton
* Black and white turtlenecks
* White sneakers
* Baseball caps
* Black, white, and khaki shorts
* Short jacket, white or basic color
* Jeans
* Swimsuit
* Swimsuit cover-up, sarong, or pareo

Chapter 9

Under It All

It won't matter that you're wearing the most gorgeous dress with matching hose, shoes, and handbag, that your hair and makeup are perfect, if your bra strap is hanging off your shoulder. The type of undergarments you choose have just as much to do with being well-dressed as does ironing a wrinkled shirt before you wear it. These are the details that matter. The details that people will never notice *unless* you get it wrong.

In Paring Down (Chapter 2), I suggested that you keep seven pairs of undies and seven bras in your drawer. That doesn't mean they have to be boring, white cotton without any feminine details. As a matter of fact they shouldn't be. It doesn't cost any more money (or very little) to buy panties and bras in colors or patterns than it does to buy basic white. It's fit and quality you're looking for. And who doesn't feel better knowing that she's wearing lacy, silky panties under a tailored suit? I know it puts a little lift in my step—it's like having a delicious secret that no one knows about but you. I also can't get away from my mother's voice whispering somewhere in my head, "What if you are in a car accident? Do you want some stranger to see you with holes in your panties?" That voice haunts me, and I feel guilty if I don't wear nice underwear.

Of course, you want your underwear to be comfortable and not noticeable to anyone else, and the latest developments in fabric and design can also help you hide bulges and reshape specific areas. These new bras, panties, and slips are nothing like your grandmother's girdles. They're comfortable, sexy, and look just like regular underwear. No one but you will know that they really contain tummy control panels or bottom lifters. Bottom lifters? Oh great, you say. *Now I'm supposed to take my big bottom and squeeze it into a panty that's going to lift it up and make it look even bigger? I'm going to have a shelf? That's just what I need.* Don't be scared of this type of undergarment or others that reshape you. They can really help. Even if you have a large bottom, a shaper will pull you in a little and reduce your jiggle. Try some on, put your clothes on, you'll see, there will be a slight difference. But buy them only if you're comfortable. I don't want you to be all squeezed in and miserable. But trust me, try them.

Bras

Is there anyone out there who hasn't tried a Wonderbra or one of its many copies yet? It seems to me—and a trip through any lingerie department will prove it to you—that all of a sudden manufacturers are paying attention to what women need and want. Size AAs now come in lacy styles instead of little-girl stretch cotton, size DDs now offer generously padded shoulder straps for added comfort. There are sports bras, bras inside swimsuits, and the return of the full slip, now with slimming panels in the stomach and thigh areas. The choice is enormous, but the chance of your finding a bra to go under any outfit is more of a sure thing. Here's how to get the right fit:

* Measure around your chest underneath your breasts and then add five inches (for odd numbers, round up) to get your band size.

* To calculate your cup size, measure around your chest across your nipples. The difference in inches between this measurement and your band size determines cup size. If there isn't any difference, you're an AA, a one-inch difference is an A cup, two inches a B, three inches a C, etc.

Bra-Less

I have been wearing bodysuits instead of bras. I tried the ones with built-in bra cups, but my breasts fell below the cups (how depressing is that?), so now I wear the cup-free styles. Yes, they flatten my breasts, but they also slim my stomach and sides. They don't leave bulges where a bra strap would be, so I feel smoother all over.

Also, I like the ones without snaps. I don't like the feel of snaps and I can never get them re-attached after I use the bathroom. They're no problem when I'm dressing, but when I'm trying to juggle a purse, and hold my skirt up, and push my jacket out of the way, they're impossible. I know, you're probably wondering if I have to take the bodysuit completely off when I go to the bathroom. I can't believe I'm telling you this—I just pull the suit to the side, sit down, and go. Hey, it works for me. ✳

✴   You still should try on many different styles to get the best fit. Sizes vary slightly by manufacturer, so a 34B in one style may fit like a 34C in another.

What Do You Need?

You need a bra to wear with everything you own. Most of your bras will be the usual style with two shoulder straps. The bulk of them should be in a smooth fabric that won't look lumpy under blouses. They can still be in colors or prints, but the fabric needs to be lace free to look right under most clothes. Now you can add specialty bras to wear with certain outfits. Buy one push-up bra (or two if you need black and white) for sexy evening wear—these are not for work if worn with a low-cut blouse. Then go through your wardrobe and see if you need a strapless bra or one that has adjustable straps to wear with halter tops, or some sports bras. If you're small, you can wear a sports bra with a flat, nonmolded front; but if you're large, you'll need the support of built-in molded cups and stabilizing straps. Try on as many as you can stand, then jog around. (Run through the lingerie department. They'll think you're nuts, but so what?) Make sure you find a style that fits and is comfortable.

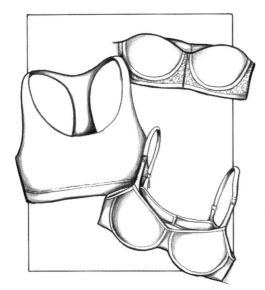

A great bra, although difficult to find, is one which has attached shoulder pads. I recently searched for one and ended up having to order it through Bloomingdale's in New York. They didn't have a sample on display, but the saleswoman knew exactly what I wanted when I asked her. I bought twenty because I am worried that they will be discontinued. Okay, so twenty is a lot, but I really love these bras. The shoulder pads are attached to the straps so they don't slip or fall down my back, and they are removable for washing. The lesson here: If you envision something in your mind, but don't see it in a store, ask. You never know.

Panties

You must try on panties before you buy them. I know, what a hassle. And you have to try them over your own panties for sanitary reasons. Panties are rarely returnable, so if you don't try them before you buy, you'll be stuck with a drawerful that you

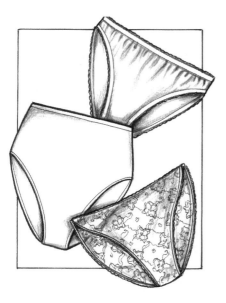

never wear or, worse, you do wear them and they ride up or show through slacks. Pick a day when you have plenty of time—and energy—and devote it to buying the right panties for your wardrobe. Look for panties that don't ride up in the rear or bind tightly around your legs or tummy. Buy one pair and take them home and wear them. If they're great go back and buy six more. I suggest starting with one size larger than the one you would normally select. For some reason, panties are sized smaller than you think. Much smaller. Even though you wear size eight slacks, you might wear a size large panty. And if you are very large, you may not find anything that fits in a regular lingerie department. It's more important to find panties that fit than to worry about having to shop in the large women's department. I know it's hard. You don't really want to buy anything that's a size large or extra-large, do you? Don't let your brain get in the way of a good fit. Tear the tags out when you get home if it helps.

What Do You Need?

If you wear slacks more often than skirts, you will need to buy underwear in smooth fabrics that won't add extra bumps and show through. Buy briefs (high-waisted) rather than bikinis to wear under slacks. Treat yourself to a few pair of lacy panties to wear under dresses and loose skirts. Make sure you buy a variety of colors (stick to off-white if you're not sure) that won't show through under certain outfits. Then fill in special wardrobe needs. Do you have that one pair of hip-hugger slacks (lucky you, if you can wear them)? Then make sure you buy a pair of bikini panties to wear with them.

Panty-Free

I have to come clean here and admit something. I rarely wear panties (I can't believe I'm telling you this. From now on, everywhere I go people will be whispering, "Is she or isn't she?") Those of you who are overweight or have thigh bulges will understand right away why I hate panties. I feel squeezed in, almost bound, and uncomfortable. I think that the bulges show through my pants. It's awful. I usually wear pantyhose under slacks, or sometimes, just stick a minipad right on the slacks and wear nothing. When I'm feeling really heavy, I wear a pair of Frank's briefs. I'm not kidding. They're roomier and don't bind at the leg. So even though you should have a wardrobe of panties for when you need them, you also need to do what works for you. ✳

Slimmers

This is where I have seen the most advances in lingerie in the past few years. Better fabrics and styles have made slimmers—or shapers—a must for every wardrobe. We all could use a little help pulling in tummies, boosting bottoms, and slimming thighs. These slimmers hold everything in place (even super-skinny women can get flabby). Voilà! No jiggling!

PANTIES: Front panels pull in tummy; separate panels in rear boost bottom.

NEW GIRDLES: Thigh-length panties help slim legs; slip with tummy and thigh panels pulls in tummy, slims thighs.

FULL SLIPS: Boosts the bust, flattens tummy, slims thighs.

TOPS: Tightens look of flabby arms.

BODYSUITS: The new ones have seamless bra cups and are made from Lycra or spandex to slim all over.

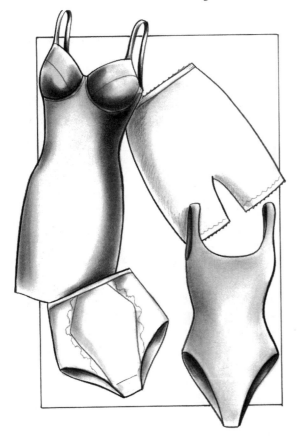

The New Colors

One area where manufacturers have really hit the jackpot is the introduction of lingerie in real skin-tone colors. This is especially good news for women of color or those with dark skin. You are not limited to black or off-white any longer. Most major manufacturers now make bras, panties, and bodysuits in nude, tan, coffee, and cocoa shades. If you get a good match to your skin tone, you will not have to worry about color showing through your clothes.

Hose

As much as we might sometimes dislike wearing pantyhose or stockings, the fact is we can't always show bare legs. If you work outside the home, chances are you will be expected to wear hose every day you wear a dress or skirt (and you should). Certainly you wear hose in the evening (right?). You need to make sure you have the right hose style and color to go with everything in your wardrobe. So you have to shop ahead and make sure you have what you need on hand. If you don't, you won't wear that great outfit you were planning on, or you'll wear the wrong color hose and ruin the whole look. You don't want to be scrambling to find the right hose five minutes before you should be walking out the door.

Please don't wear a dark skirt with white hose. Or a white skirt with black hose. Your hose or tights should have equal value (not too bright, not too pale) with your wardrobe. Fuchsia, purple, and red hose are just too bizarre. They're for teenagers. If you just can't decide, you're safe wearing sheer hose that let your natural skin color show through.

A word about sandals: If you wear hose with sandals or open-toe shoes, don't wear those with a reinforced toe. You think you're saving money because your toes won't poke through the hose, but really it looks so silly. Make sure your nails are trimmed neatly instead.

What Do You Need?

How many pairs of hose you need really depends on how often you wear them and how quickly you go through them. You need your basic everyday hose to match your basic wardrobe, so you can wear them with everything. If you wear hose every day, buy them by the dozen. Many department and hosiery stores offer a free pair with every dozen or some other bonus for regular customers. For during the week, buy durable hose. Those that contain Lycra or spandex (please, not the shiny kind) will last longer and keep their shape all day long.

Now go through your wardrobe and make a list of the other hose you need to go with spe-

Girdle Be Gone

I shied away from the new body slimmers because I still have nightmares about wearing my first merry widow (bra, girdle, garter belt, all in one). I wore a strapless dress to a prom in high school. We went to dinner before the dance and by the time we got to the prom I could barely breathe. I called my mother to ask her what to do. (I was having gas pains from my neck to my bottom. I literally couldn't stand up.) She told me to take it off. I did, and buried it in the trash can. I never wore a tight girdle again. But I do now wear thigh slimmers (they make some that go all the way to the ankle) and butt lifters. They are so comfortable and make a difference in how my clothes look. Give 'em a try. ✳

cific outfits (take them to the store with you if it's a hard match). I always buy at least two pair of any hose—just in case. Also, once you've gone through all the trouble of finding the right color, you might as well stock up. Colors are discontinued all the time, and then you'll just have to search again.

It's not always so easy to determine the right size. Each manufacturer sizes just a little bit differently. Ask for help, read the chart on the back of the package, and take them home. Try one pair before buying a bunch (and do buy a bunch if you find the perfect pair). If they don't fit, take them back. It's not your fault if the package sizing isn't accurate.

One Last Word

I can't possibly tell you how to shop for the type of lingerie you wear in the bedroom. It's your fantasy time. It's more of a feeling and what you feel comfortable wearing. I will say, though, treat yourself. Don't obsess about it. You can be a sex kitten, a little girl, a femme fatale. Whatever you can imagine. Don't be afraid. He'll adore it. He won't think it's silly. Give him a thrill.

If the person you share your bed with insists on buying you lingerie that you hate, either wear it a few times to make him happy, or, better, ask to go shopping with him so you can choose outfits together. That can be a very sexy shopping trip and open a whole new world for the two of you.

Ban White Hose

I have a thing about white hose. I suppose there are times when they look okay, although I can't think of one. They almost always make legs look pink—especially on women of color. And who decided that a navy blue dress is perfect with white hose? Unless you are heading out on active duty, it looks silly.

I once ran into a client—who knows how I feel about white hose—who was wearing them. I screamed, "What are you doing!" and she knew exactly what I meant. I actually dragged her into a drugstore and made her buy a different pair and change in the rest room. Right then. That's how much I hate white hose. ✳

Chapter 10

Expressions

I have to confess something here. We are now at the chapter I love the best. I love accessories. They are my favorite, favorite things. I love my accessories, I love my friends' accessories, their friends' accessories. I would probably love your accessories. I couldn't put myself together without them. Probably the most important thing I could say is that you shouldn't, either. They are the single thing that will tell the world who you are. It's not a dangerous obsession to have. The best part is that accessories can be *cheap*, yet make you look like a million bucks.

With the right accessories you can fool people into thinking that you have an extensive wardrobe when you really have only a few good outfits. When I was first starting out as an actress I had to go and see casting agents every day. Often I would visit the same casting directors over and over again until they decided who to book for the job. Since I was still on a very limited budget, I had only a few nice things to wear. I couldn't wear the same thing every day . . . but I did and no one knew it!

I went out and bought a very nice black suit (my basic suit). It had a jacket and a skirt . . . nothing fancy. I also bought a few blouses. Then I went to work. I dressed in the suit and took the extra blouses in a bag and went shopping. I bought scarves, pocket squares, pins, and belts that turned my one suit into many different outfits. Because I was wearing the suit I could see what worked right away. That's one of my great secrets. *Always* wear the outfit you are trying to perk up when you go to buy the accessories. It makes sense, right? But you wouldn't believe how many women don't do it. They buy belts and pins and scarves that they think will work with the outfit, and then get home to discover that they don't work at all. So the accessories—and the outfit—get pushed to the back of the closet and forgotten. Does this sound familiar? Are you smiling? Come on . . . you have to agree that it is a total waste of money—and time—to buy things you don't wear when you could be buying things that make your wardrobe sing.

Once you acquire a good collection of accessories it is important to keep them organized. My accessories are categorized and stored neatly in my closet. So neatly that I always tease my mother about shopping for accessories in the "Linda Dano Boutique." She dresses and then visits my accessory store to complete her look (of course she always looks great). I gave you some storage ideas in Chapter 2: Paring Down, and I'll give you more here.

Not everyone needs to have or wear every type of accessory. For instance, you may not like hats. That's okay. Concentrate on the extras that you do like; the ones that tell people who you are. Still, read through this entire chapter; you may actually find things you like and want to try. Please, keep an open mind.

You're probably wondering right now, *What exactly are accessories?* Okay, let's start with a list:

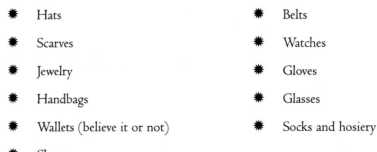

✳	Hats	✳	Belts
✳	Scarves	✳	Watches
✳	Jewelry	✳	Gloves
✳	Handbags	✳	Glasses
✳	Wallets (believe it or not)	✳	Socks and hosiery
✳	Shoes		

Now that you know what accessories are, let's figure out what you need and why. Most women go into a department store and blow right past the accessories. You don't even see them. You head right for the clothes as if the scarves and belts and pins are on another planet. You shouldn't. Take one, just one, afternoon and devote it to investigating these departments. Just see what's there. Try things on. Find out what you like and then come back with a few outfits to accessorize. Okay, just one outfit to start. Come on, I'll take you on a tour.

Hats

Hats are not for everyone, or maybe you just think that. If you've never worn a hat, it will take a while to become comfortable with even the idea of wearing one. If you are shopping for your first hat, start with one that is small brimmed (wide brims should really only be worn at the beach or at a summer garden party). It could be felt. It could be cotton. Or knit. But it must be in one of your four colors (you might choose your basic color and then add a ribbon or flower or a pin in one of your other colors); it has to match what you wear.

Wear your hat perched just above your eyebrows. If you wear your hat pushed back on your head you'll just look dopey, not chic. And if I see you on the street, I'll run over and tug it down if it's pushed back. Truly I will.

Many of you probably don't wear hats because you are worried about "hat head." That's what happens to your hair after you've been wearing a hat for a few hours. There are two solutions to hat head: One, find a hat so comfortable you can leave it on, making it a part of your outfit; or, two, carry a small brush and a travel-size bottle of styling gel and disappear into the ladies' room to fluff up your hair.

Once you buy your first hat, it will be easier to buy more. When you buy a new outfit, make yourself go to the hat department and try a few on. Select styles you wouldn't normally try, like a pillbox or a knit beret (the best thing about knit hats is that they can be shoved into your purse and pulled out for a hair emergency). You may not go home with a new hat, but you've taken the first step. Bravo!

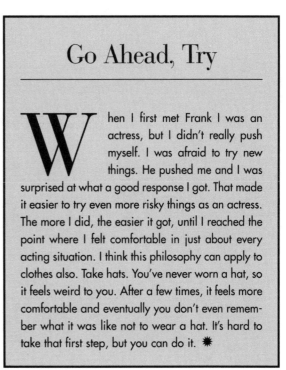

Go Ahead, Try

When I first met Frank I was an actress, but I didn't really push myself. I was afraid to try new things. He pushed me and I was surprised at what a good response I got. That made it easier to try even more risky things as an actress. The more I did, the easier it got, until I reached the point where I felt comfortable in just about every acting situation. I think this philosophy can apply to clothes also. Take hats. You've never worn a hat, so it feels weird to you. After a few times, it feels more comfortable and eventually you don't even remember what it was like not to wear a hat. It's hard to take that first step, but you can do it. ✳

TO STORE: Store hats either in their boxes, alone on a shelf, or on a hat rack. (That's what I do. I love to look at them all lined up.) Be careful with them. Once they lose their shape, forget it. They won't look good and neither will you.

Scarves

Scarves are what I consider your most important accessory. They add so much style to even your basic suit that you could wear the same outfit every single day, with just a change of scarf, and look completely different. That doesn't mean you can go totally nuts and buy any scarf you want. You still have to stay within your four colors so that the scarf matches everything you own. But you can buy solids to go with a print jacket, prints to go with solid jackets, or even prints to go with other prints. You can buy oblong scarves that hang down to your jacket hem or you can buy squares that knot around your neck. There are a million combinations that can look great; you just have to experiment.

My favorite type of scarf is an oblong made from chiffon (this can be a silk chiffon or a synthetic chiffon). Pure silks and polyesters tend to slip and slide out of place. Chiffon has just enough nub to help the scarf stay put. *Here's a trick:* Fold scarf in half lengthwise; wrap around neck; pull loose ends through loop at fold and pull tight; tuck ends into blouse top. Voilà! I guarantee that the scarf will stay put all day long.

For square scarves I like to fold them in half to make a triangle, then roll them up tight and tie in a small knot at the neck (sort of like a necklace). Remember, it's just a touch of color you're looking for. This style will also stay put all day.

These are just a few ideas. If you buy a scarf in a good department store, the salesperson can give you more ideas on how to wear it. Ask. You can wear scarves any way you like, as long as you do wear them. You don't have to buy expensive 100 percent silk scarves to make a chic fashion statement. I have seen great scarves for as little as $6.99 on sale. It's the look and feel that are important, not the price. Buy a bunch . . . and wear them.

I consider pocket squares to be part of the scarf family. A pocket square tucked into a jacket pocket adds a lot of style for pennies. You don't even have to buy an actual pocket scarf. You can go to a fabric store and buy twenty-five cents' worth of fabric, bunch it up, and tuck it in a

It Has to Be You

I once had a client at Strictly Personal who had seen someone else wear a really big scarf over a suit and decided she wanted to try that look, too. She bought the scarf and brought it over to try on at my house. We got her all wrapped up in the scarf, and she looked okay. But she kept adjusting it here and there, trying to get it to feel right for her. I told her it looked good and that she could add it to her wardrobe. Later that day, I happened to run into her on the street. She was still adjusting the scarf and, boy, did she look uncomfortable. She said that it wasn't working for her. It looked right, but she didn't feel right. It didn't fit with her personality. I told her to return it. She did, and that was the right decision for her. Remember, you don't have to wear everything you see. ✳

pocket. You don't have to finish the ends because no one will see them. I have three evening pocket squares that are just pieces of fabric. I change the buttons on my jacket to shimmery ones, tuck in a pocket square, and I've transformed a plain black jacket into an evening ensemble.

There are a couple of styles of scarves that I couldn't live without for winter:

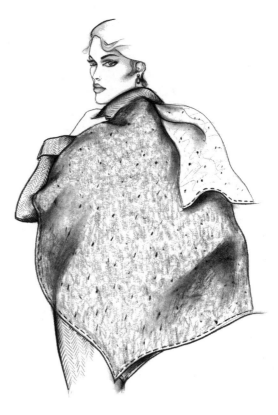

ADVENTURE SCARVES

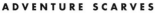

These are big, really big, scarves that you can wear loosely folded over your shoulders or wrapped around your neck a few times.

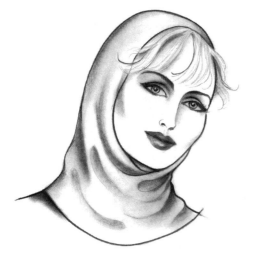

COWLS

These are really hats that look kind of like a tunnel. You pull them over your head and scrunch up the bottom around your neck. You put your coat on after the cowl for a nice, finished (and warm) look.

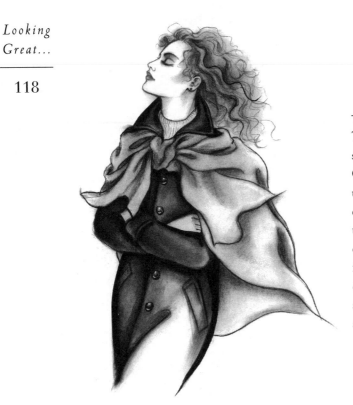

LONG SHAWL

There are two types of long shawls that I wear all the time. One is a winter, wooly one that I use as a coat during the fall and early spring and over my coat in truly cold weather. The other is one in some kind of shimmery fabric to wear over evening clothes. You can even make this to save money. It really dresses up a simple black dress.

TO STORE: Good scarves usually come with their own boxes. I recommend refolding and storing in those boxes. For all others, either fold neatly and place on shelves, or drape from hooks. If you use hooks, don't pack them in; they may get lost. Find a space that has a little room around it to keep scarves from wrinkling.

Jewelry

There are two kinds of jewelry: serious jewelry and fun jewelry. The serious stuff is jewelry that you buy (or someone buys for you) because it's the real thing. It is real gold, platinum, or silver, has real stones, and usually costs a ton of money. You have to know what you're doing to buy serious jewelry. What's in your jewelry box is a very personal thing. You don't need all of this, you may need none of it, but if you truly want a good starter collection, here's what to buy:

Earrings

* small gold or silver earrings
* small cultured pearl earrings
* half-carat diamond studs

Necklaces

* cultured pearls, any length you like
* gold or silver chain to hold interchangeable charms

Bracelets

* gold or silver bangles (solid rounds), as many as you like
* gold or silver open weave (like a charm bracelet)

Watches

* basic watch with black or brown leather band; face should be gold and silver tone to match all jewelry
* evening watch; maybe a thin gold or silver band, a diamond face, an antique

Extras

* wedding band (good for you!)
* engagement ring
* a cameo pin (especially an antique one)

The above list will cost you thousands of dollars, and you may not wear good jewelry all the time. Just about everything on that list can be bought as fakes. Trust me, no one will know the difference between diamonds or cubic zirconia or Diamondique. *I* can't even tell the difference. It's all a matter of what you like. What you feel comfortable wearing.

Accessories are really the place where you can give into trends. Especially jewelry. Mass-market department stores have reams of costume jewelry at reasonable prices. If long, hanging earrings are in, you can buy them; if strands of faux pearls are the rage, you can buy those, too. You can buy whatever is in season, and next year buy all new accessories. You'll have them forever. Your size may change, clothes go out of fashion, they wear out, they take a lot of space to store. Jewelry can last forever. If it goes out of season, it's easy to store. Don't worry, it will come back in style again. Someday. It always does.

TO STORE: Serious jewelry belongs in a safe or a safety-deposit vault at the bank. All of your other jewelry has to be in a place where you can see it and get to it easily. I store mine in clear Lucite jewelry boxes that have little compartments for each piece. I have one box for earrings, one for necklaces, one for bracelets, pins, etc. I stack them on top of one another in a drawer. I can take out the whole box and see everything at once. Nothing gets lost or separated from its mate this way. Also, jewelry doesn't get dusty since these boxes have lids.

Handbags

You of course already have your basic everyday handbag and a good evening bag in your basic color. Where to go from here? I happen to be one of those people who change handbags every day, so I have a lot. I keep all of my important things in a smaller bag that I can easily transfer to my daily handbag. You, too, can have many bags if you really love them. And use them. And store them properly.

There are millions of styles out there, and new trends are being started every day. If you have $4,000 to spare you can even buy an Hermès Kelly bag. But why? I have found great bags and backpacks at Kmart for under $20. You shouldn't spend a lot of money on a bag that you know is a trend bag. (You should spend more on your basic bag that you use often.) You will look just as chic and hip with a trendy $20 bag as with a $200 trendy bag. You'll only use this "in right now" bag for a few months, so don't waste your money on it. Put the money into something that will last, like upgrading your basic jacket.

I think one bag you do need is a sturdy tote for all of those things you carry around that won't fit in your handbag. Buy a leather or tough canvas tote in your basic or bright color. Empty it and clean it about once a month. How long has it been since you've looked in the bottom of that thing?

TO STORE: Storage depends on how often you use each type of bag. If most of your bags are the seasonal or special occasion type, consider buying an under-the-bed storage box. Stuff bags with tissue paper, fold soft handles inside and snap shut. Place them in a box, or if you have the shelf space, line them up on a shelf (without cramming them in). Evening and smaller bags can be hung from hooks installed on the back wall of your closet.

Shoes

I consider shoes accessories. They can make or break an outfit. You will never go wrong wearing one of your basic pairs (pumps, loafers, evening pumps), but it's more fun to match shoes to different outfits. That doesn't mean you should go crazy buying tons of shoes you'll never wear or buying shoes because you're too depressed to buy clothes. It's about finding your style through shoes. Finding that perfect pair that really *adds* something to your clothes.

If you need some guidance, here are my ideas on the next few pairs you should buy after your basic three:

* Spectator pumps or flats in your basic color and white

* Boots in your basic color (Height depends on body type. See Chapter 3.)

* Lace-up flats to wear with slacks (can be patent leather or other fun style)

The problem with shoes is that they eventually wear out no matter how well you take care of them. One of the things I've learned over the years is that if I buy a pair, wear them, and find I truly love them, I have to go back and buy another pair right away. If I don't, they will have been discontinued by the time they wear out. For some reason if I alternate wearing the two pairs, they last longer than if I wore one pair until they wore out and then switched to the other. I don't know why this is, but it is. Often I even buy the same shoe in another color if I really love them.

We all love sales, me included. Or I should say, me especially. I have learned, though, to be very cautious at a shoe sale. We think, *What a great bargain! I can't pass this up!* But sometimes you should. Shoes should fit perfectly as soon as you try them on. Unlike clothes, you can't have them altered. You may think (or hope) they'll stretch, that you'll wear them in, etc. That's not going to happen. If they hurt when you try them on, they'll hurt when you wear them (although you probably won't because they're so uncomfortable). It's worth it to pay full price to get a good fit.

TO STORE: You can store shoes in a telescoping low rack at the bottom of your closet, in an over-the-door shoe bag, or in their original boxes stacked on a shelf. See Chapter 2 for full details.

Belts

Beyond your basic ones, belts can be like jewelry. They can add a little flash to an otherwise plain outfit. One belt changes the whole look. (Those with thick waists, skip over this section, belts are not for you.) The only real rule about belts is that the buckle has to match the tone of your jewelry: gold jewelry—gold belt buckle; silver jewelry—silver belt buckle. The only exception is if you are mixing silver and gold jewelry. Then it doesn't matter what tone buckle you have.

After your basic belts, add these:

* chain belt that sits at waist

* chain belt that sits at hips

* leather belt with interchangeable buckles (then you can just buy new buckles)

* lamé or velvet evening belt

I also love to hang things from my belts as an additional accessory. Little change purses, silver trinkets, a pair of gloves, really anything that can hook on and that appeals to me. You can make your belt more of a fashion statement and more you by using a little creativity. Try it.

Gloves

Gloves have really fallen out of style as an accessory. I live in a cold climate, so in the winter I really need them. It's easy to pull on any old warm pair you can find, but it's a lot more fashionable to make them a part of your look. Of course you need your basic wool pair, or leather if you can afford it, in your basic color, but after that go for colors or prints or whatever says you.

For evening, gloves make a very elegant statement. They can be long or short, cotton or silk. They look fabulous with a sleeveless dress. Two things: Never wear jewelry over gloves, and remove them while eating.

Glasses

For those of you who wear glasses, you probably have one pair that you wear until they break or your prescription changes. Glasses are expensive so I understand that you can't have a whole collection, but it's important that you find a pair that complements your face and your wardrobe. Frame color should match one of your four colors, not your hair or skin tone. The same rules go for sunglasses (although you can probably buy a few pair since they're less expensive).

Choose the frame style according to the shape of your face.

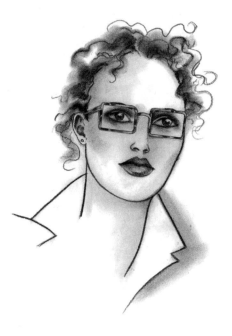

Oval

Many styles look good on an oval shape face; best is square with slightly rounded corners.

Round

Look for frames equal in width to the widest part of face. Glasses with brow bars make face appear longer. Rectangular is best shape.

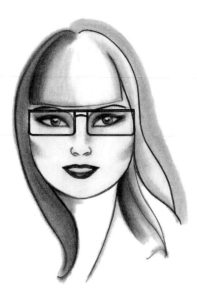

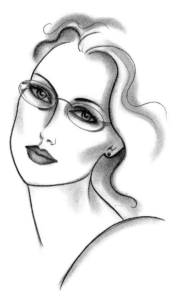

Diamond

Frames should not be wider than cheekbones. Oval frames—or even rimless—are best.

Square

Frames should be as wide as face. Oval frames are best.

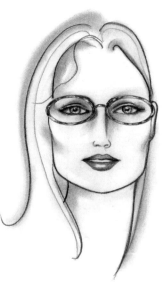

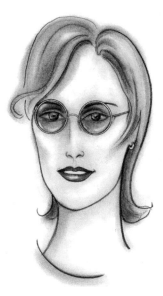

Oblong

Frames should not be wider than face. Round or square frames are best.

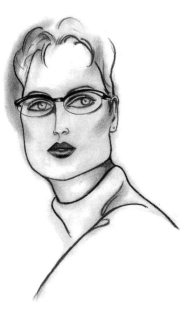

Triangle

Frames should be wider than face. Unusual shapes (like cat-eyes) work well. Metal frames with rimless bottoms work, too.

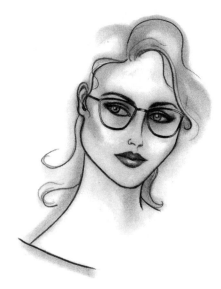

Heart

Frames should not be wider than forehead. A rimless style or frames that drop toward bottom are best.

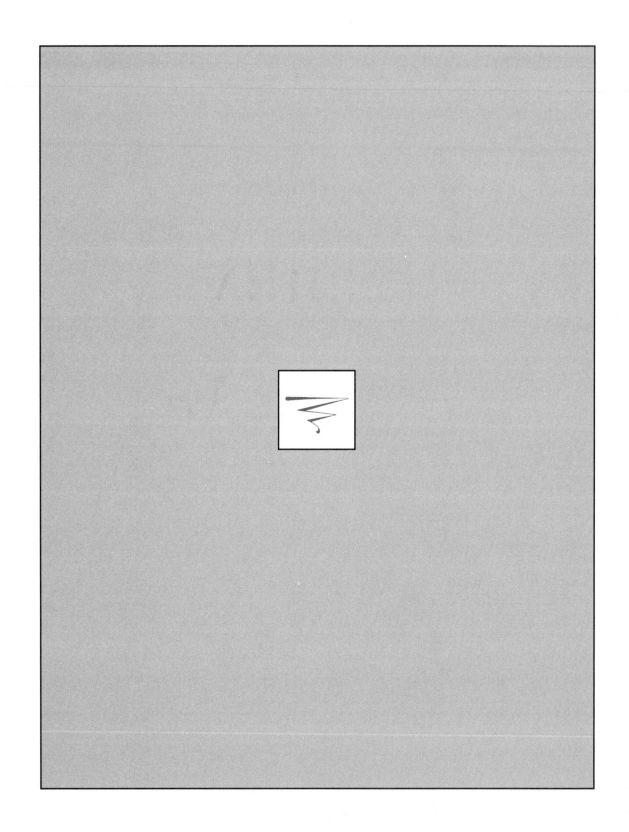

Part III

Beauty

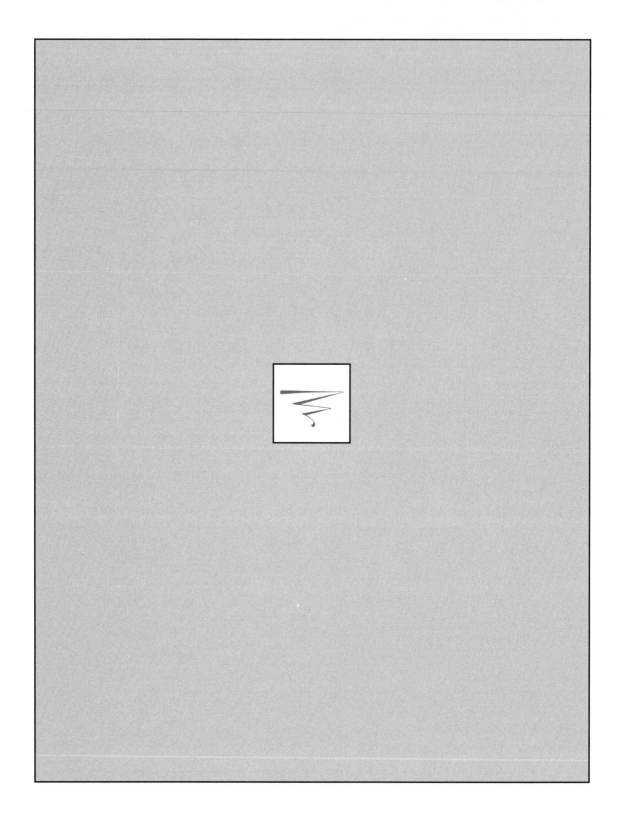

Chapter 11

Makeup:
The Final Accessory

You can't expect to look well-dressed without makeup. I know . . . it's a pain in the . . . but, you have to trust me on this. Not only will you look better, you'll feel better, too. The hard part is that you have to learn *how* to apply the makeup that is going to make what you have look its best. That takes practice and frequent updates. But mostly practice. As you age, the type and colors of makeup you wear will have to change. Fashion and the times also dictate changes. Sometimes it's hard to tell what works and what doesn't. You may think you look great because you're used to seeing the same face and applying the same makeup you always have. You get stuck in an age. Sometimes it takes another opinion to convince you to change. It happened to me, and I should know better!

I was cohosting the *Attitudes* show on Lifetime, and the show was doing very well. I was cruising along, thinking that everything was perfect. A great career on *Another World,* a loving husband, and now a popular talk show. One day there was a knock on the door of my New York apartment. I opened it to find all of the producers of *Attitudes.* They came in and proceeded to confront me on a very sensitive issue. It was like those drug interventions when the offender is trapped in a roomful of friends and forced to admit he has a problem. They said, very seriously, "Linda, it's about your makeup. We need to help you change it." Well, I was floored. I had always worn the same makeup (see, that's what I'm talking about), since the sixties. Oh. That was the point, the producers said. "This is the eighties—it doesn't work anymore."

I fought them tooth and nail, but eventually came around to trying new things. And you know what? They were right. I looked ten years younger and felt prettier than ever. Since then, I make sure to get expert advice every now and then, and I'm less afraid to try new things. I have an advantage. I ask my studio makeup people for advice; if I'm doing a talk show or a personal appearance, I ask those makeup stylists for new tricks; and I go to department stores—like what I want you to do—and ask the women who work there for help. We all need experts to help design a makeup routine that works for us. I can't tell you, here in this book, that you should wear black eyeliner on your upper lids if you're a brunette. I'd have to know what shape your eyes are, what shape your face is, what you're wearing today, etc. Makeup advice is something that has to be done in person, hands-on.

What I can do to help you is to tell you what all the different makeup products are and what they are used for. So that's what I'll do. I'll show you which makeup brushes are best, how to store (and discard) your makeup, and how to remove the new semi-permanent lipsticks . . . yes, they do eventually come off. This will be like your own personal tour of a cosmetics counter. I can also tell you the tricks I've learned from makeup artists—professionals, who apply makeup all day long.

Foundation

WHAT IS IT? Foundation is used as a makeup base to even skin tone and fill in small lines. It comes in liquid, stick, and cake forms. For sheer all-over coverage liquid works best. Cake and stick foundations offer heavier coverage, but can often look too heavy and unnatural. There is also a product called dual-finish foundation. It comes in a compact case and looks like a powder. You can use it as a powder, to touch up foundation or set makeup throughout the day, or you can wet it with a damp sponge and apply like foundation. I use a stick foundation, which is very thick. I know how to apply it lightly, but unless you can, stay away from it. Foundation shouldn't look like a mask.

HOW TO BUY IT: It is extremely important that foundation color match skin tone. If it's too dark or too light it will look unnatural and be impossible to blend at the neck line (and this is *very* important). This is the one makeup product for which it pays to get expert advice in choosing the right color for your skin. Go to a salon or department store makeup counter to try different shades. Try it on your face, not the back of your hand. Go to every counter if you have to. They don't charge you just for asking questions. Be wary of bad lighting; ask to take a small mirror outside (even if the counter lady has to go with you) to double-check the color in natural light. Many cosmetic companies, such as Prescriptives, will mix colors for individual skin tones. This is a bit more expensive, but you'll get a perfect match.

You may need to spend more on foundation than other makeup products, but it is so important. It is the base for all of your makeup. If you choose the wrong shade or the wrong type, you'll never look good. This isn't a splurge; it's a necessity.

Foundations come in different formulations for different types of skin. If you have dry skin (do you even know what kind of skin you have? ask at the cosmetics counter), look for a foundation that contains a moisturizer; if you have oily skin look for an oil-free product. Many also contain sunscreen.

HOW TO APPLY IT: Use a makeup wedge sponge (you can buy these in any drugstore). Run sponge under clean water and then squeeze out excess water. Pour a small amount of makeup in the palm of your clean hand and dip sponge (or with cake or stick types, wipe a small amount on sponge). Start with small areas—around eyes, lips, nose—and then blend to cover entire face. Blend carefully around hairline and neck.

WHEN TO DISCARD IT: Why am I telling you this? You haven't even bought the damn stuff yet, and I'm telling you how to get rid of it! It's because bad makeup is not good for your skin and you need to replace it every once in a while.

Foundations last about two years. Oil-based products might separate, so shake before using. If product does not remix after shaking or ever has a foul smell, discard and buy a new one.

Concealer

WHAT IS IT? Concealer is used to hide blemishes, but also to highlight or reshape features. It is a thick, creamy product. Also, you know those green, yellow, and pink sticks they're selling now? The package says if you have red skin tone, use the green concealer under your foundation to cover it, etc. Forget these. Your natural skin tone will still show through, except now you'll look like you have an extra layer of makeup on.

HOW TO BUY IT: Concealer usually comes in stick form. You can buy it in your local drugstore; any brand will do. Choose a shade one color *lighter* than your skin tone. Now be careful here; don't buy concealer that's too dark.

HOW TO APPLY IT: Concealer should be applied before foundation, not after. It can be applied right from the tube or using a makeup wedge. Dot on blemish (go lightly; too much makeup highlights blemishes) and then blend with make-up wedge.

    Trick: For under-eye circles, your first thought might be to cover puffy area entirely. Don't. This only highlights the area. Instead, draw a line of concealer on the indentation below the puffy area to fill in gap. Puffiness will disappear.

WHEN TO DISCARD IT: Concealer lasts a long time, but if it begins to flake or separate, toss it and buy a new one.

Highlighter

WHAT IS IT? Highlighter is just that, a product to highlight and reshape features. The product is not labeled "highlighter," it is just a darker-color loose powder or blush.

HOW TO BUY IT: Buy highlighter in one shade darker than your foundation. Highlighter should be brown, not red. Loose powder works best and is easiest to apply. You can choose the shade yourself and buy a less expensive drugstore brand or go to a cosmetics counter for expert advice.

HOW TO APPLY IT: Highlighter should be applied with a large powder brush in big sweeping strokes before applying blush and after foundation. This is really tricky. You have to have a very light hand. More is not better. It is most commonly used to sweep a line below regular blush to create a more prominent cheek shape. Start from your cheekbone and brush back to hairline. Blend. Blend. Blend. When you go for your makeup application lesson—and I know you will—you'll learn other places where highlighter can be applied to enhance your features.

    Trick: As women age, the jawline and neck lose definition. Mine sure have. There's only one way to really get rid of a double chin . . . chop, chop. But you can give yourself a mini-makeup face-lift by brushing highlighter along jawline and then in a triangle from your outer jaw to about three inches below chin. Really *blend edges.*

WHEN TO DISCARD IT: Powder highlighters should last forever if you keep them in a dry place. If moisture makes product clump, it's time to replace. Cake or blush products last about two years.

Powder

WHAT IS IT? Loose powder is what you use when your entire makeup application is complete to set makeup for the day. Loose powder is translucent, which means it has no color. It reduces shine and soaks up excess oil. It also keeps foundation from seeping into skin creases and caking up.

HOW TO BUY IT: Powder can be purchased at your drugstore or cosmetic counter. It's really a matter of feel; find one that you like. It's hard to make a mistake.

HOW TO APPLY IT: Use your large powder brush and apply sparingly. Remember, powder is used to set makeup, not add to it. Re-powder throughout the day if skin is oily or shiny.

WHEN TO DISCARD IT: Loose powder lasts a long time if kept dry. If it begins to clump, buy new.

Blush

WHAT IS IT? Blush is used to add color and definition to cheeks. It comes in powder, liquid, and cream form. Powder offers the easiest application and most natural look. Liquids and creams are very difficult to blend, so I don't recommend them. I can't even use them and I've had a lot of practice. I always end up looking like a clown when I use liquid blush. It must be a secret that people conspired to keep from me. I'll stick to powder, thank you.

HOW TO BUY IT: Blush is all about color. It should always have a soft rosy tone: too-bright colors make you look garish; too pale and why bother? You can buy blush at the drugstore, but only after you've gone to a cosmetics counter and tried out the samples. I suggest buying your first blush in a place where you can practice application, and then to save money, replace by matching with a cheaper brand. Many cosmetic companies will custom-mix a color for you. Remember to view in natural light before buying.

Blush is the hardest thing for me to buy. I'm never happy with the color no matter how many I try. I'm dark, so I wear a brownish-tone blush. You'd think this would be easy. It's not. It's even hard for me to find the perfect tone of blush for my skin. I think I come close, but I'm still looking for the perfect shade.

HOW TO APPLY IT: Most blush products come with a small brush. Don't use it. Always apply powder blush with a large blusher brush, using big sweeping strokes from cheekbones back to hairline. Use sparingly. Blend edges using brush or make-up wedge.

Trick: In a pinch you can use powder blush as eye shadow. Apply with a sponge-tip applicator or makeup wedge, then blend.

WHEN TO DISCARD IT: Blush lasts about two to three years if stored in a dry place. Replace when powder begins to flake apart or looks oily.

Eye Shadow

WHAT IS IT? Eye shadow is used to add color and definition to the eyes. It comes in a large variety of forms from powder to cream to pencils. It also comes in every color imaginable. I am not like most women: I don't own a full palate of colors, and I don't think you need to, either. Those huge trays of colors sold at bargain prices are really tempting, but you need to limit yourself to the colors that work for you.

I don't care who you are, you should never wear big patches of blue or purple or green on your eyes. Here's where reading too many magazines can get you into trouble. You see all the models wearing bright eye colors. Why can't you? Because you can't. You'll look silly. Maybe a teeny line of blue next to your eye, but that's it. Your eye shadow should be like your basic color. Pick a brown or gold or russet, or mix them together. Remember, eye shadow is to make you more beautiful, not make you look garish.

HOW TO BUY IT: It's really hard to go wrong when buying eye shadow (it's the application that causes problems). It's not expensive and you can afford to buy many shades. First decide the type of product that's easiest for you to use and apply.

Powders look more natural and are easier to blend; creams and pencils look shinier and require a finer touch.

Go to the cosmetic counter at your favorite department store and have a professional apply eye shadow for a daytime look, and then ask her what she would add for an evening look. If you like the colors she has chosen, ask if they are available in a package (all the colors together). If not, you'll have to buy separate packages. Again, the first time I would recommend buying what the professional suggests, then replace with drugstore products when you run out. I buy those three-in-one packages in the drugstore.

HOW TO APPLY IT: Eye shadow should always be applied with a sponge-tip applicator, makeup wedge, or an eye-shadow brush (unless you're using a pencil, in which case, apply directly, then blend with wedge or sponge-tip . . . are you confused yet?). Sponge-tip applicators will apply the heaviest coating of shadow, brushes the lightest. (Eye shadow should be applied before eyeliner and mascara). Start with the lid section closest to the eye and work up and out. I know you've already gone to a professional who has taught you which colors to use and how to apply them, right? If you haven't, get going. Then practice, practice, practice. You didn't learn to ride a bike in one day, you won't learn to apply makeup quickly, either. You have to work at it.

Trick: To avoid having eye shadow gather in creases of lid, apply loose powder (with a brush) first, and then apply eye shadow over it.

Trick: For close-set eyes, don't apply shadow all the way to inner corner of eyes. Start at about the edge of your iris and work outward. Darker colors on outer edge will widen eyes.

WHEN TO DISCARD IT: Powder eye shadows last just about forever, as do pencils when routinely sharpened. Creams tend to separate. When a cream looks flaky or oily, discard.

Eyebrow Pencil

WHAT IS IT? An eyebrow pencil is used to fill in empty sections of brow or to extend them.

HOW TO BUY IT: Choose a shade slightly lighter than your natural brow color. You can feel safe picking out a color on your own and buying at the drugstore.

HOW TO APPLY IT: Eyebrow pencil should be used sparingly—less product than you think is needed. You don't want to look like Groucho Marx. The goal is to fill in and define, but also to achieve a natural look. Don't buy a pencil without a sharpener; the pencil must be sharp when applying. Starting in the center of your brow (the part that looks the darkest), use small, light strokes, to fill in gaps. Then go over brows with an eyebrow brush to blend and smooth. You can also use a clear eyebrow gel to set brows in place.

Trick: You can also use a matte brown eye shadow to fill in gaps in brows. I do this all the time; I prefer it to a pencil. Fill in using a fine-tipped brush and then use an eyebrow brush to blend.

WHEN TO DISCARD IT: When regularly sharpened, eyebrow pencils will last forever.

Eyeliner

WHAT IS IT? Eyeliner is only for those with very steady hands. It is used to line the eyes to create definition. It comes in both liquid, pencil, and cake forms, none of which is particularly easy to use. It can be done, but it takes practice.

HOW TO BUY IT: Eyeliner can be purchased at the drugstore. It comes in dark colors like black, brown, and dark blue. You will definitely want to get advice from a professional before deciding if it's right for you at all. Eyeliner is used more for evening than during the day; it adds a little glamour.

HOW TO APPLY IT: Pencils are the easiest to use and will produce a softer, smudged line. Liquids and cakes should be applied with a fine brush. Liquids are ready to use right from the bottle; for cakes, wet brush and then coat with liner. Apply above eyelashes on upper lid, and if you're really steady, under lashes below eye. (Never apply on lower ridge next to eye, above lower lashes. Product will irritate eye.) I use a liquid eyeliner that comes with its own teeny, tiny brush. I apply a straight line and then smudge the edges a little with my finger for a softer look.

Trick: As we age, our eyelids start to droop. This makes eyes lose definition and depth. Use an eyeliner pencil to draw a light line just above your natural eye crease, then apply eye shadow over it. This will give the illusion of a wider eyelid and less droop. Be careful, go very lightly, practice this. If you get it right, it will give you an instant eyelid-lift.

WHEN TO DISCARD IT: Cakes and pencils (when sharpened often) will last two to three years. Liquids may separate and need to be tossed sooner; always rinse brush after use and before replacing in bottle to prevent bacteria from entering product.

Mascara

WHAT IS IT? Mascara is a product used to coat and define eyelashes. If you use only two makeup products everyday, I would recommend that they be mascara and lipstick. Both are easy to apply and add a lot of punch for time spent applying.

HOW TO BUY IT: Mascara comes in dark colors (you can buy light blue and purple, but don't) like blacks, browns, and dark blues. It also comes in many formulations: waterproof, water-soluble, with added moisturizers, with lash thickeners, etc. What you really need is an inexpensive drugstore product that goes on smoothly and has an applicator you feel comfortable with. Waterproof *will* smudge if you get it wet and then rub your eyes (but is still tough to completely remove). Moisturizers make mascara smudge more. I use water-soluble. It's still pretty tough, but it comes off with soap and water.

HOW TO APPLY IT: Mascara should be applied only with the applicator it comes with. It should be the last product you apply before you set your makeup with loose powder. Use eyelash curler *before* applying mascara. If you get clumps, gently comb them out with a lash comb. Apply to upper lashes with smooth upward strokes. Many makeup artists do not recommend using mascara on lower lashes; if you do, use only one coat. If it smears on skin, apply a small amount of makeup remover to a cotton swab and wipe mascara off.

Learning from the Pros

I get my makeup done every day on *Another World,* so I am always in a position to learn about new products and how to apply them. That's why I urge you to go to a professional for a consultation, whether it's at a makeup counter or a salon. The women who dispense this advice live with makeup every day and know what works. One of the best tips I've gotten came from Melanie Dimitri, who does my makeup on *World.* She uses a silicone primer on my neck and eyelids before applying foundation and eye shadow. This product is made by many cosmetic companies but for some reason doesn't get a lot of attention. It looks like a moisturizer. What it does is fill in some of the little wrinkles and give the skin a moister look. As we age, skin—especially on the neck—tends to dry out. This makes it hard for makeup to adhere properly. The silicone base helps makeup stay smoother and last longer. ✳

Trick: For truly thick lashes, apply a light coating of loose powder to lashes, then apply mascara. Wait until it dries, then add a second coat. Comb out clumps.

Trick: I use a light-brown mascara as an eyebrow tinter. I wipe applicator off on a tissue and then use light strokes through eyebrows. You have to apply very lightly to do this correctly.

WHEN TO DISCARD IT: Because the mascara applicator comes into contact with the eye, bacteria is then transferred back into tube. Replace mascara every six months to keep fresh.

Lipstick

WHAT IS IT? Lipstick adds color, evens out lip color, and can even help change the shape of your lips depending on application. It is the most important makeup product. In my opinion, you should never be without it. If you wear no other makeup, lipstick will at least give you some color on your face.

HOW TO BUY IT: There must be thousands of lip-color products. Lipstick comes in tubes, pencils, pressed into compacts, you name it. They come in matte, glossy, creamy, iridescent. The colors are also endless. If you stick to drugstore products you can probably afford to buy as many as you want. Department store cosmetics are often twice the price so you may be more limited in your collection. By all means get a professional's advice before choosing colors for your skin tone. The key is to find a lipstick that feels and looks good on your lips; you won't wear it if you don't feel comfortable in it. Sometimes the taste of a lipstick ruins it for me, and I can't wear it even if I love the color.

HOW TO APPLY IT: It's really hard to go wrong if you follow your natural lip line, smack lips together, and blot with a tissue. If you are trying to change the shape of your lips with lipstick—and that's one of its great attributes—you will need a professional's advice first. Lipstick can be applied directly from the tube or pencil, or with a lip brush. Be very careful with semipermanent lipsticks and lip stains; once you apply them you will need a special remover product to get them off.

Trick: To make regular lipsticks stay put longer, apply lipstick, blot, then reapply. You can also use a lipliner pencil as a foundation: Apply liner all over lips, then apply lipstick on top. This is what my makeup artist does on Another World.

WHEN TO DISCARD IT: Hopefully you'll be using lipstick every day and will run out before it needs to be replaced. For seldom used colors, a year is a good rule of thumb.

Lipliner

WHAT IS IT? Lipliners do two things: They prevent lipstick from seeping into fine lines around mouth and help reshape lipline if needed. The product is very similar to lipstick, but in a waxier formulation. It comes in pencil form. You can also use a darker shade of lipstick to line lips, but I think a lipliner works better because it is a thicker formulation (lipstick tends to leak into small cracks around mouth).

HOW TO BUY IT: Your lipliner should be *slightly* (not much) darker than your lipstick. If it's too dark it will look like a tattoo. You can buy it anywhere; more expensive is not necessarily better.

HOW TO APPLY IT: Lipliner should be applied from the pencil or with a brush (if you're using lipstick as a liner). Draw a thin line around outer edges of lips (use the flat side of the pencil for a softer look) and apply lipstick over it.

Tricks: To add fullness, draw a line of pencil just outside natural edge of lips. Trace shape of bow on top to maintain natural look (a straight line will look clownish); use a lip brush to fill in lipstick and blend edges of liner. Add a dot of lipstick one shade paler (gold tones work well) to center bottom lip for extra fullness.

WHEN TO DISCARD IT: Lipliner pencils last forever if regularly sharpened.

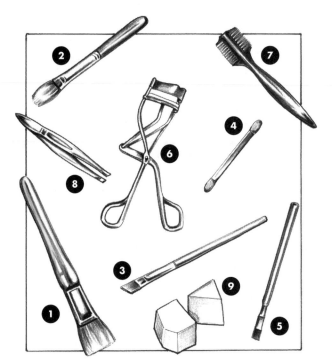

Essential Tools

1. LARGE POWDER BRUSH
Use with powder to set makeup.

2. BLUSH BRUSH
To apply powder blush.

3. EYE SHADOW BRUSH
To apply powder eye shadow.

4. SPONGE-TIP APPLICATOR
To blend eye shadow, highlighter, or concealer.

5. LIP BRUSH
Use to line lips or fill in with lipstick.

6. EYELASH CURLER
To curl eyelashes; use before mascara application.

7. EYEBROW BRUSH AND COMB

To shape eyebrows.

8. TWEEZERS

To pluck eyebrows.

9. MAKEUP WEDGE SPONGES

To apply and blend foundation or cream blush and eyeshadow.

Shaping Brows

Eyebrows frame your most important feature: your eyes. Their shape and texture can determine the look for your whole face. You can have a professional pluck your brows, or have them waxed, but with a little practice you can easily do it yourself.

To determine natural brow shape hold a pencil alongside your nose next to your eye. This is where your brow should start. Swivel top of pencil to line up with outside corner of eye. That is where your brow should end. Then looking straight ahead, line pencil up with outside of iris. This is where your eyebrow should reach the height of its arch.

To pluck:

* Hold a warm washcloth over brow area for a few minutes to soften skin.

* Use a magnifying mirror and begin plucking with a pair of slant-tip tweezers. Grab hair at base and pull firmly in direction of hair growth. Pluck hairs between brows first, then move to brows themselves.

* Pluck a few hairs from each brow, then go to the other one to maintain evenness.

* Less is more. Do it slowly. Wait a day then pluck some more. Remember it takes a long time for new hairs to grow in.

Taking It Off!

I wear lots of heavy makeup every day, and I have to take every speck off to avoid damaging my skin. Sometimes this is a chore I feel like skipping, but I know I can't. Luckily there are plenty of removal products on the market to help. Maybe too many products. How do you know which one to buy?

I read the labels and use the products for the places they are made for. Eye-makeup removal products are formulated to remove mascara, eyeshadow, and eyeliner. The one thing I really watch out for are added fragrances and botanical oils. These ingredients can irritate the eyes and really make allergy sufferers pay for using them. To be safe, use a product that contains mineral oil as the main ingredient. It won't bother eyes and will remove the toughest waterproof mascara. Apply by soaking cotton pad or ball (make sure it's cotton; many drugstore brands are rayon—check labels!) and gently wiping, using new cotton balls/pads until they come away clean.

I use a gentle facial cleanser to remove foundation and any dirt that sticks to it. This is an individual choice. If your skin is oily, choose an oil-free preparation. If it's dry, choose a cleanser that contains a moisturizer. Apply by putting small amount in palms of hands and then smoothing over face. Place hands on face and then pull away, creating a sucking motion to pull makeup from pores. Repeat a few times. Rinse with clean water until makeup is removed. (I know I'm not supposed to finish up by using soap and water, but I can't help myself. I love the feel of really clean skin.) Finish with an application of toner on a cotton ball or pad to tighten pores and remove last traces of makeup. Face is clean when cotton ball/pad comes away clean.

The new semipermanent or nontransferrable lipsticks present a true challenge to remove. The only thing that works are products made to remove them. Right now only a few companies make them (try department-store cosmetic counters), but I have no doubt that with the popularity of these new lipsticks, they will soon be manufactured by everyone.

The Easiest Manicure and Pedicure

For a truly finished look you have to have polished fingernails, and in the summer toenails. This doesn't mean you have to wear attention-getting bright-red polish or have dagger-length nails, just that nails have to be clean and trimmed, and at least a coat of clear polish. You look really silly with gold stars or little pictures painted on your nails; keep it simple. Follow these easy steps for a quick manicure and pedicure:

Manicure

1. Wash hands and scrub nails with a nail brush.

2. Clip or file nails into a squarish shape, rounding corners slightly (this shape is less prone to breakage).

3. Buff nails with a nail buffer and then rub hand cream into nails, cuticles, and hands (for real softness, heat a towel in the microwave for about thirty seconds and wrap around hands for about three minutes).

4. Push back cuticles with an orange stick wrapped in cotton—never cut. Do trim any hangnails.

5. Apply a clear base coat (not needed for pale polishes because they won't stain nails). and let it dry completely.

6. Apply two coats of color (if you can't wait for each to dry, apply one and then go do something; come back later and finish).

7. Apply top coat, let dry. You can then apply a sealer product if you choose.

8. Dip an orange stick wrapped in cotton in polish remover and clean up any wayward polish. Allow nails to dry completely before using them.

Pedicure

Most of us never take the time to really pamper ourselves. A pedicure is that kind of indulgence. Few people will see your artistry so why bother? Because it's for you. You'll know. It's a treat for *you*.

1. A pedicure is for your entire foot, not just the nails. Soak feet for about fifteen minutes in soapy water (use bath oil or gel) to soften skin.

2. Use a pumice stone or file to smooth calluses and remove dead skin.

3. Cut toenails straight across. Too-rounded edges can cause ingrown toenails.

4. Rub a huge helping of moisturizer all over feet and then gently push back cuticles with an orange stick wrapped in cotton.

5. If your toes are a little twisted, separate with foam pads or tissue. Paint with base coat. Let dry.

6. Apply coat of color polish. Let dry. Apply second coat. Let dry completely before applying sealer (if you want) or fast-drying topcoat.

Chapter 12

A Good Hair Day

I hate my hair. You hate your hair...I know you do. I don't know a woman who doesn't hate her hair. If it's naturally curly, like mine, you dream of straight hair. If it's stick-straight, you wish for just a day of bouncy curls. If you're a brunette, you want to be a blonde. Every woman thinks her hair is the worst of all. (It isn't, mine is!) So what can you do about it? Lots. First of all, you have to look in the mirror and say, "Okay, this is me. This is who I am. I may not like it, but what can I do to live with it and make myself look and feel better?" That said, you have to start to investigate different strategies for turning unruly or limp locks into an easy-to-care-for style that makes you feel confident about your looks. That's what this chapter is about: Making *every* day a good hair day.

I grew up with long, out-of-control, curly, wavy hair. When I first became a model in the sixties I spent hours straightening my hair. I ironed it, brushed it to death, and did everything I could to make sure it was stick-straight. Of course, one quick rain shower and it was back to its usual tricks. I spent so much time on my hair, and yet I still really loathed it. That is, until one day when I was sitting in my agent's office and I overheard a conversation from the booking desk. A client, Curl-Free, was looking for a model for a TV commercial. They wanted someone with super curly hair that they could apply their product to and straighten. I jumped up and ran over to the desk and said, "What about me? I have curly hair." Well, they hadn't ever seen me with curly hair because I made sure they never saw me unless my hair was ironed to perfection. "No, no," they said, "there's no way your hair could be curly enough." So I ran home, washed my hair, stuffed it into a big hat and ran back to the agency. They were shocked, but agreed I might book the job. Guess what? I did! Of course, that day I loved my crazy hair. And I really started to accept what I had and learned to style it in many different ways to suit my mood or job prospects.

There are a couple of things I had to learn about hair before I could really begin to love—well, okay, *like*—my own hair. Here are two of the most important things you have to understand about hair before we can move on: First, whichever type of hair you were born with—straight, curly, thin, thick—that's the type you are always going to have. You are not going to wake up one day and all of a sudden have a different kind of hair. No matter what you do, what you put on it, it's still going to be the same hair. That's not to say that you can't *look* like you have a different type of hair, just that you will have to work at it every day if you truly want to control curls or create thickness. This chapter is all about working with what you've got, which brings me to the second major point about hair: It's dead. D-E-A-D, dead. As soon as a fresh sprout leaves the safety of your scalp, it's dead. Really, really dead. The longer it grows the more time it has to be swinging around dead. And getting more and more damaged. So you have to take care of it to prevent the kind of damage that can't be fixed.

You know all those ads for hair products that claim to "bring more life into your hair" or "revive damaged hair"? It sounds good, but forget it. Dead is dead. No product—even those made with live placenta (I swear they make one)—can make hair live. Because why? Come on, say it. It's dead!

The Cut

How your hair is cut is the single most important factor in how it looks. You have to find a good stylist whom you trust. I don't care if you have to go to five before you find "the one." It's so important. I can't tell you in a book which cut is going to work for you. A stylist will evaluate your hair type, face shape, and your lifestyle, to determine what will look good on you. You can bring pictures of cuts that you like, but a good stylist will nix them if they honestly will not work in your hair. Here are some tips to finding, and working with, a good stylist:

✳ Get references from friends.

✳ Ask the stylist about her training. How long has she been working? How long has she been at that salon? Has she taken a recent course in coloring, perming, new styles? Salon owners are often the best choice (although hard to book) because they will have the most experience and really want to please you.

✳ On your first appointment go with your hair in its natural state. Don't curl it or use hair spray. The stylist needs to see and feel your hair as it is.

✳ Be honest. Tell the stylist how much time you can spend on your hair every day. If you like to wear it up, tell her. If she suggests a style that you aren't sure about, speak up. If when finished, you aren't happy, explain why and ask her to try and fix problems right then.

✳ Don't leave with wet hair. Many salons charge extra for blow drying, but you need to see the style dry before you decide if you like it.

✳ Ask her to explain what she's doing so you can achieve the same style at home. Is she using a special type of brush which you don't have at home? What styling product is she using?

✳ If after a few days you realize that you aren't happy, or you can't style your hair like the stylist did, make another appointment to explain the problem. A good stylist will fix problems free of charge.

✳ If you're truly not happy, speak to the owner. Owners can't make changes unless they know what the problem is.

What Is Hair?

Here's what's going on with your hair: You have about 100,000 strands of hair at any one time. New ones are coming in all the time and old ones are falling out. The hair inside your scalp is living inside little follicles. As soon as it pushes through the scalp it dies. You grow new follicles all the time. So if you lose one hundred hairs a day, new ones will soon replace them.

Once the hair is outside your scalp it begins to deteriorate. The outside shell of each hair shaft is called the cuticle. The cuticle is what protects the cortex and medulla, the inner layers of each shaft. The health of your cuticle is what determines how your hair looks. Everything you do to your hair—shampooing, brushing, drying, curling, perming—has the potential to tear off small pieces of the cuticle. When the cuticle is damaged, your hair will look dull and limp; if it's really damaged, the cortex and medulla will break down, too, and you'll get split ends or serious breakage. Once the damage occurs there is nothing you can do to permanently restore a hair shaft. The good news is that you can use conditioners to fill in the missing cuticle pieces to protect hair and have the appearance of shiny, healthy hair. Of course, the best option is to not damage the cuticle in the first place. For starters, you should shampoo, dry, and brush hair gently. Then, try to limit processing (perms, coloring, etc.) because the more you do to your hair, the more damaged it becomes.

Shampoos

The purpose of shampooing your hair is to clean it. The basic ingredient in all shampoos is detergent, which attracts and lifts dirt off your hair. Anything else is added only to improve the feel or smell of the product. Nonetheless, hair product manufacturers continue to market shampoos labeled with promises to correct every hair problem imaginable. Some claim to fix sun-damaged hair, permed hair, oily hair, brittle hair, dry hair, etc. Then there are those for oily hair, normal hair (what's that?), those that claim to add protein, or fix the frizzies. Very few of these claims can be met, yet we all continue to search for some magic formula that is going to transform our hair. Here's why that's not going to happen: All shampoos are made up of about 70 to 80 percent water; they all contain about 8 to 10 percent detergent; which leaves about 10 percent for all of the remaining ingredients. The remaining ingredients are usually fragrance or some kind of emollient to give you smoother hair *while* you're shampooing. They do nothing for the permanent condition of your hair. The thing about shampoos is that they are meant to wash out of your hair; none of the ingredients remain on your hair after washing. As a matter of fact, you *should* rinse thoroughly to remove all of the detergent.

So what shampoo should you use? Really, any brand will do. You don't need to spend $15 for a tiny bottle of shampoo if a $3 bottle of a

A Pro Tip

Annette Bianco, my hair stylist on *Another World*, has given me some great hair tips over the past fourteen years, but the best is probably this: Have an idea of the type of style you are trying to achieve, but don't set it in stone. Be flexible and willing to take it in another direction if that's where your hair is headed that day. Hair reacts to the weather, the type of shampoo you use, even to the water you use to rinse it with. If you are away from home, chances are all of these elements will come into play. Sometimes you just have to go where your hair takes you, even if it's not the style you had in mind. Try it—it may be better. ✳

drugstore brand will do the same thing. Ask your stylist what she would recommend for your type hair. Don't ask her for a brand name (although I'm sure she'll suggest her salon's product), ask her what ingredients will work best for your hair, whether your hair is oily, dry, permed, damaged, etc. You really have to go on feel. If you like the smell and feel of a shampoo, that's what you should use. Don't buy based on price. Expensive is not necessarily better.

How often you wash your hair depends on how dirty it gets and how much natural oil is in your scalp. In the end it doesn't really matter how often as much as how: Put a quarter-size blob of shampoo in your hand, rub hands together to spread shampoo. Apply to scalp and then use fingertips to gently scrub scalp (it's often not necessary to scrub bottom of hair at all). Rinse thoroughly to remove all shampoo. Directions on shampoo bottles always say "Repeat." Trust me, there is no reason to wash hair twice (other than using up more shampoo so you have to buy more) unless you've just dumped your head in a vat of tar.

Conditioners

Conditioners contain ingredients that *are* meant to stay in your hair after rinsing. But they don't create any permanent changes in your hair. Not permanently anyway. They won't make it thicker or make it grow faster (no product can make your hair grow faster). What conditioners do is fill in the missing pieces of cuticle that have broken off due to brushing or processing (perming or coloring). They make hair appear shinier and fuller because they adhere to the hair shaft, even after rinsing. You should thoroughly rinse after conditioning because the ingredients that are meant to stay in hair will; the excess will wash out. There are products called "leave-in" conditioners that you do not rinse out, but they have to be used sparingly and carefully. Too much will weigh hair down and may even make hair feel sticky. You should use a shampoo labeled "clarifying" every few weeks to rid hair of excess conditioner buildup.

Conditioners also make hair easier to comb, which results in less breakage to cuticle. Again, your choice should be based on feel, not price. If you like the smell and how your hair

Static-Free

Nothing irritates me more than when there is static in my hair. It happens mostly in the winter when the heat is on (it drys the air). Hair is flying around and you get a shock every time you touch something. I have a little trick I use to control static: Use Static Guard. (Most women use it to unstick skirts from pantyhose.) It comes in purse-size cans. Spray on your comb or brush and run through hair. You can also use a static-free dryer sheet and just rub on hair. Hey, it works! ✳

looks, that's the conditioner for you. Expensive salon products are not always the best for you. Experiment.

Styling Products

Mousses, gels, and sprays are used to help hold style in hair. Mousses are the lightest and spread through hair easiest. Gels are a little thicker and should be used sparingly. Too much will weigh hair down. Revitalizers are almost all water and can best be used to perk up a style at the end of the day. Sprays hold hair in place after styling. All of these products are useful, but they are all pretty much the same. Ask your stylist which ones are best for your type of hair. Again, ask for ingredients, not brand names. The most expensive products often contain the exact same ingredients as the cheaper ones.

Coloring

Long gone are the days of heavy single-process hair coloring, which could only be done in a salon. The newer coloring products can easily be applied at home and rarely result in catastrophe. A careful reading—and following—of the instructions is essential, but really, anyone can color her or his own hair. Here are descriptions of the products currently on the market:

TEMPORARY HAIR COLORS: These products come in the form of shampoos or dyes. They will add subtle color changes to hair (they will not cover big swatches of gray) and work well to camouflage new growth until you are ready for an all-over dye. These products work better in lighter hair than dark and will last through a few shampoos.

SEMIPERMANENT HAIR COLORS: These products stay in hair through about ten to twelve washings and will change color slightly (not large patches of gray). They do perk up color and give it a shinier appearance. Great to cover new growth until you are ready for an all-over dye.

INTERMEDIATE HAIR COLORS: These are actually permanent dyes, which stay on hair until you cut it off (the package may say they last through twenty-five shampoos, but they really never wash out). The difference is that the colors are more subtle so you won't notice new growth as much. They change color one or two shades and cover a good amount of gray (if you are totally gray, you have to use a permanent dye).

PERMANENT HAIR COLORS: These products can change your hair to any color you choose and will last until you cut your hair off. They will also cover all gray hair. New growth will be very visible unless you recolor roots. Permanent dye needs to be reapplied about every four to six weeks depending on rate of new growth. I like permanent dyes because they coat the hair and make it look shinier.

HIGHLIGHTS: It is very difficult to highlight (add streaks of color to) your hair at home and achieve a natural look. Unless you are very, very experienced, this is one process that is best left to a professional.

Perms, Curls, and Straighteners

You have straight hair; you want curls. You have curls; you want straight hair. We all want our hair to be different. The good news is that it can be. It takes some work, and a very good stylist, but it can be done. The current perm and straightening solutions are more gentle than those of the past and when applied correctly result in a natural look.

All perm and straightener solutions work the same way. They contain chemicals (some advertise as "botanical," but they still create a chemical reaction) which break down the structure of the hair, and depending on the type of rods (rollers) used, then seal in a new structure. The chemicals teach your hair to behave in a different way and hold it that way for about two to three months. The perm will eventually relax and new growth will appear, creating the need for a trim or touchups. You absolutely need to go to a trained stylist if you are always going to perm or straighten your hair. The constant assault of chemicals and processing can damage hair and a professional will work to minimize the damage. I know people who perm their own hair, but I could never do it. If you are only perming every now and then for a different look, it's probably safe to use an at-home kit (the solutions are not as strong as salon solutions, so it may not last as long).

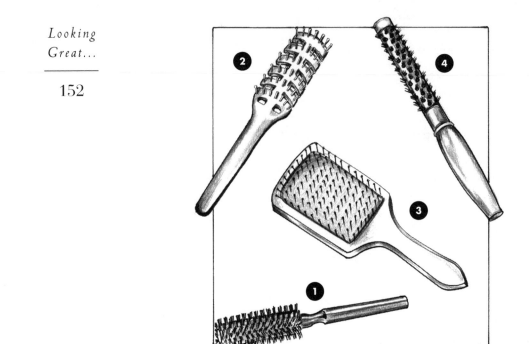

Hair Tools
Brushes

1. ROUND BRUSH
To create flips and add body to straight hair.

2. VENT BRUSH
For blow-drying. Vents let air through to hair.

3. PADDLE BRUSH
Best for long, straight hair. Brushes without pulling.

4. HEAT-RETAINING BRUSH
To style hair. Metal core stays warm and works like a curling iron.

Blow Dryers

I bet every one of you uses a blow dryer. If not for styling, than at least for drying wet hair. It's probably the one hair appliance found in every household. It can be a terrific styling tool. It's easy to use and hard to do real damage. Of course, if you use a blow dryer to dry and style your hair every day, you will cause damage simply because you are handling your hair often. Pulling wet hair with a brush while blow-drying will surely break off some of the cuticle. Here, then, are some tips for getting the most from your dryer:

* Pre-dry hair before styling. Either let hair air-dry a little or use a strong blast of cool air to pre-dry roots before styling (flip head over and dry roots from bottom).

* If you have super-curly hair and you are trying to straighten it with a blow dryer (you may be better off having it professionally straightened to prevent daily damage), dry sections around face first. These sections tend to be curliest and also dry fastest.

* Height at the scalp is what makes hair look fuller, healthier. To get height, either use one of the new blow dryers with a "finger" attachment, or use this brush technique: Place brush about two inches from your scalp, bristles down. Push bristles into hair and then push brush toward the part, creating a little "bridge." Hold and dry. Move to the next section.

* After hair is mostly dry, use a brush to create style. Give hair a blast of hot air to soften, hold in brush and then switch to cool air (before removing brush) to set style.

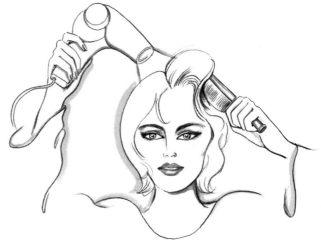

* To prevent frizzies, hold dryer about eight inches away from scalp. This distance helps keep cuticle flat, which will make hair look shinier.

* Use brushes with natural bristles for blow-drying. Plastic and nylon bristles can cause static.

* For an end-of-day lift, spritz hair with water, flip over, blow-dry.

Curling Irons

Curling irons come in many sizes and strengths. The best ones come with a variable temperature control (low temperatures do least damage to hair) and a tip that doesn't get hot so you can hold it with your other hand while wrapping hair. The larger the barrel on the iron, the larger the curl will be.

Since curling irons can only be used when hair is dry, you must first blow-dry, adding an extra step to styling your hair and one more chance to damage it. For this reason, I suggest using curling irons to style hair on the second day after you wash it (if you don't wash every day). Spritz hair with water, blow-dry for a few seconds, and then curl. Try not to use a sticky styling gel or mousse before curling; it will make hair stick to the iron and damage it.

A great alternative to a curling iron is a hot-air styling brush. It's a combination blow dryer/curling iron. A great benefit is that you can use it on wet hair, eliminating one step in your styling process. Hot-air brushes are great for straightening and smoothing out curly hair.

Hot Rollers

With the advent of curling irons and hot-air brushes, hot rollers have lost some popularity and many manufacturers no longer make them. That doesn't mean that they aren't useful, only that few of us have the time to dry and roll hair every day. Hot rollers are best for long hair that would take just as much time to curl using a curling iron. By the time you're done rolling one side, the other side is finished. For short hair, a curling iron is quicker. They are also great for adding lift to top of hair (use when hair is dry, otherwise get lift from blow dryer).

Hair Straighteners

Electric hair straighteners look like two paddles put together with metal plates on the inside. They are essentially an iron that you close around hair, one inch at a time, and pull down. Straightening hair this way takes forever. (I know, I used to do it.) I would strongly recommend having your hair professionally straightened instead of using one of these every day. The constant assault of heat and pulling on the paddles can really damage hair much more than the straightening chemicals used in a salon.

Chapter 13

Skin Deep

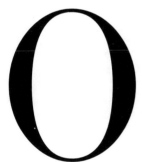kay, let's get right to it...I'm fifty-three (and fifty-four is just around the corner—May 12, 1997). I don't look so bad, do I? I've been lucky, that's for sure. I still have relatively nice skin. I've been blessed with good genes. That part is inherited and can only be attributed to pure luck. But I know that another reason my skin is still healthy and young-looking is that I have always hated lying in the sun. It's probably because I'm a type-A personality and couldn't sit still . . . or maybe it's because I'd always rather go shopping. But thank goodness I never damaged my skin. Long before anyone even knew the damage that overexposure to the sun could do, I was ahead of the game. So even though I grew up in a place where the sun shines almost every day, I managed to hide from it pretty well. It's a good thing, too, because no one used sunscreen in those days. A deep, bronze tan was considered healthy-looking . . . and sexy. The boys liked it. . . . *I* liked it. I still like it, but I don't tan because I know I'd have to pay for it in the end.

My mother had a friend who just lived in the sun. Her name was Ellen, and I loved her dearly. As I grew up, she grew leathery. Many years passed when I didn't see Ellen, and when I did . . . boy, did she look awful. She looked old. She looked very tired and very unhealthy. It scared me, and it was then that I knew the damage that the sun could do. I had seen the proof.

So there are two factors that determine how your healthy your skin looks: one, heredity; and two, exposure to the elements like the sun and pollution. But that doesn't mean that just because your mother and grandmother have wrinkled, tough-looking skin, that you will, too. Genes do play a role, but we now know so much more about protecting our skin than we did when they were younger. We *can* change the course of hereditary skin damage. Many new products—both prescription and not—also help hide some of the damage you've already done.

There are a gazillion products and treatments on the market for use on the skin. Go to any drugstore and you will be assaulted with an entire aisle of moisturizers, lotions, toners, cleansers, acne treatments, soaps, scrubs, and a whole section of "miracle" products that promise to get rid of your wrinkles. (Let's get one thing straight: no gel, cream, or lotion will erase wrinkles permanently. I don't care what they promise, it just can't be done.) Do you need all of this stuff? Probably not. Should you buy it? Probably not. But as long as you stay on the inexpensive side and it makes you feel good, go ahead. First read on to learn what these products are and how they can help your skin.

First: Protect

The one and only way to have healthy skin is to protect it from damage. (Okay, so you can have a face-lift, but it's less painful and cheaper to halt damage before you get to that step.) The biggest offender to the skin is the sun. Not only does it dry skin and create wrinkles, it can also lead to skin cancer. Those of you who have had a lesion chopped off your nose know it's not a pretty sight. So why take chances? It's so easy to protect skin these days. Tons of moisturizers and foundations come with a sunscreen right in them so you can easily apply with makeup every morning.

One of the biggest falsehoods is that you are only at risk in the summer when the sun is shining. Ultraviolet radiation (often abbreviated as UVA and UVB rays) is there year-round. And even on cloudy days, the rays still penetrate and burn your skin. UVA rays penetrate the skin deeply and cause wrinkles, while UVB rays cause sunburns and skin cancer. To protect against both you need to wear a suncreen and a hat.

With all the products and strengths of sunscreens on the market it's hard to know which to choose. Make your decision based on how long you plan to be in the sun, but use at least a SPF (Sun Protection Factor) 15. That means you can stay in the sun fifteen times longer before you burn than if you were not wearing sunscreen at all. Most people with normal skin will begin to burn in about twenty minutes, depending on sun strength that day. Apply sunscreen all over *before* you get dressed (or just on face and neck if you are going to be indoors most of the day) to avoid missing areas close to shorts or swimsuit lines. Reapply after swimming or if you are sweating. Even if the product says it's waterproof, reapply anyway.

Since sunscreens come in so many forms—gels, lotions, sprays—and strengths, it's still hard to know which to buy. All types will cover and protect the same way, so if you like the feel of a lotion, use that (see, that part's easy). As for brand, here's a tip: Expensive is not necessarily better. The basic ingredients in all sunscreens are the same. You can pay more for packaging and advertising if you want, but why? Also, you may feel inclined to use less if the product was very expensive. Sunscreen only works if it's liberally applied, so buy a cheaper product. You'll use it more often and gain all the benefits sunscreen can offer.

Faking It

Okay, so you've smartened up and said goodbye to sunbathing forever. That doesn't mean you have to suffer lily-white skin, too. You can have the appearance of a healthy tan year-round thanks to the advances in self-tanners. Gone are the products that left you with orange, just-been-through-radiation, streaky legs. The new products go on so smoothly and evenly that no one will know your tan is fake. It takes a bit of practice to learn to apply correctly—and also some testing to find the right product and color—but the results can be terrific. Here's how to apply:

✳ Rough patches may soak up tanner differently, resulting in a blotchy finish, so before applying, use a loofah or rough washcloth to exfoliate skin. If you still have some rough patches (usually around knees and elbows) apply moisturizer to those areas before applying tanner. Wait about 15 minutes before applying tanner after exfoliating.

✳ Test the product on a small patch of skin for two reasons: one, to make sure it will not irritate skin; and two, to check color.

✳ Apply sparingly. You can always add color; you can't take it away.

✳ Start at toes and work up to avoid rubbing color off on your arms while applying the self-tanner to lower body.

✳ Apply in even strokes (circular strokes work well to make sure tanner is absorbed by skin in every direction) and really rub in well. If your product is too thick and doesn't rub in well, mix with some moisturizer (this will also lighten color).

✳ Wash your hands thoroughly when done, paying special attention to in between your fingers. Use an old towel to dry hands; tanner may come off on the towel.

✳ Wait until tanner is completely dry (about fifteen minutes) before dressing.

A couple of other self-tanning products are worth mentioning, and using. Tinted moisturizers are great. You can use them instead of foundation for even coverage. Even better is a tinted moisturizer that also contains a sunscreen. You can't beat three-products-in-one.

Also good are bronzers. They usually come in powder form (although there are some creams for the very brave). Apply with a blush brush to cheeks, forehead, nose. These are the areas that the sun would naturally color so bronzers can give you that sun-kissed look without the sun damage.

The Promised Land

In the past ten years dermatologists and cosmetic companies have combined forces to produce a whole array of new products which promise to eliminate wrinkles. Many, like Retin-A, were originally developed to fight acne and were then discovered to also halt wrinkle production. Formerly only available by prescription, some retinoids—such as retinol, retinol acetate, and retinol palmitate—are now available in products sold over-the-counter. Here's the latest news about Retin-A, Renova, and alpha-hydroxy acids:

Retin-A

Retin-A is a derivative of vitamin A and is available only by prescription (cost is about $15 per month, depending on your pharmacy). You must see a dermatologist before use (don't use if you're pregnant or nursing). Retin-A works by causing the skin to shed its older, outermost layer and then replacing the exfoliated cells at a faster rate. The effect of this is the appearance of fewer and less deep wrinkles. The new skin growth looks fresh, clean, and younger.

Retin-A is available in different strengths. The higher strengths may cause stinging, itching, or burning; hence the need to be under a doctor's care. It can also dry out skin, although use of a moisturizer will help combat that problem.

Retin-A does not permanently get rid of wrinkles. It must be used continuously. If you stop use, the wrinkles will reappear. Also, during use of Retin-A, skin is very sensitive to sun and you *must* wear a sunscreen under makeup everyday. You must also follow your dermatologist's instructions for use.

Renova

Renova is the new kid on the block. It works very much like Retin-A (and costs about the same) and is also only available by prescription. Renova is not an acne medication; it is prescribed to halt damage from the sun. The main difference between Retin-A and Renova is that Renova is formulated in an emollient base, making it more moisturizing. Renova has not been studied as extensively as Retin-A, but small studies have shown that it produces less stinging and burning.

As with Retin-A, you must continue to use Renova to reap its benefits. Once you stop, skin will return to its previous state. When in the sun you should wear sunscreen and a big hat to protect skin from further damage. (Renova also makes skin more sensitive to sun.) Also, follow your dermatologist's instructions for use.

Alpha-Hydroxy Acids

If you haven't heard of alpha-hydroxy acids (AHAs) you must be living on a different planet. They're the skin-care news of the nineties. AHAs are derived from glycolic, lactic, citric, and malic acids. They make the skin look fresher and younger by peeling off the outer layer of dead skin cells and stimulating growth of new cells.

AHAs are found in every type of skin-care product on the market, from moisturizers to cleansers to masks. All of these products are available over-the-counter and come in many different strengths. You need to check the ingredient list to determine just how much is in the product you use. Most over-the-counter products contain less than 2 percent AHAs. That strength is fine to moisturize but will not come close to the effects of Retin-A or Renova. A product needs to contain 8 to 15 percent AHAs (these products will be more expensive) to be really effective in softening wrinkles.

Choose one product that contains AHAs for your skin-care routine. A moisturizer is the best choice because it stays on the skin; cleansers wash off. Don't use more than one AHA product; you could really irritate your skin. To apply, wash your face, wait fifteen minutes for skin to stabilize, and then apply AHA product.

Get into the Routine

In order to have and maintain healthy skin you must take care of it. That means establishing a routine that includes cleansing, moisturizing, and occasionally treating yourself to a deep-cleansing facial. Doesn't this sound like a lot of work? Whew, I'm tired already. Really, you don't have to make your skin-care routine into a big deal which involves sixty-five products (that you never use) sitting on your bathroom counter. If I can help you understand what all of these products do and why you should use some of them, you can pare your routine down to about five minutes a day. I should say here that after I take my makeup off (see Chapter 11: Taking It Off!), I love to scrub my face with soap and water. I know it's very drying—and against all the rules—but I love the squeaky-clean feel it leaves behind. Like I said earlier, I was always protected from the sun and I've been blessed with good genes, so I don't feel bad about this one indulgence. It works for me. That's what this whole book is about: learning all you can and then choosing the things that work for you. I can help with the learning part.

Cleansers

Starting each day with a clean face and body is essential to feeling good. If you feel sticky and grungy, there's no way you can feel confident about your appearance. Those with dry skin may need only a quick shower and a dose of moisturizer to prepare for the day. Those with oily skin may need a deeper cleansing with a special facial cleanser to remove oil. Believe me, there are products out there for everyone. How do you know what kind of skin you have? And which product to use? Basic skin-type guidelines are:

* Dry Skin: Feels tight and rough; dry patches often appear.

* Very Dry or Sensitive Skin: Prone to tightness and discomfort of dryness and sensitivity. Many products irritate skin.

* Combination Skin: Both oily and dry. Usually forehead, nose, and chin are oily and shiny.

* Oily Skin: Prone to breakouts and blemishes, enlarged pores, and a never-ending shine.

These are only basic guidelines. You may find that a product designed for oily skin only makes your skin more oily. If I had very dry skin or very oily skin, I would go to a dermatologist and ask him or her to prepare a cleanser in the office for my use at home. This is one of the services that dermatologists offer, but which very few women know about. They are experts at choosing ingredients that work well for your skin. It's well worth the cost (many insurance plans cover this anyway).

Whether you use a product (and I think the fewer products, the better for your skin) or soap and water to clean your face, you should also scrub gently to remove dead skin cells. On face, use a washcloth; on body, use a loofah or rough sponge. Pat dry and then wait fifteen minutes before applying moisturizer or makeup.

Moisturizers

Talk about product overload. There are hundreds of moisturizers on the market. They range from $1.59 drugstore brands to $75 department-store jars. The job of moisturizers is to prevent dry skin and therefore wrinkles. Once you have wrinkles, no product in the world will completely eliminate them. If you see a product that promises to get rid of wrinkles, it's lying. It's that simple. Don't buy that product because it won't work (and besides, who wants to support a liar?). It really, really won't work.

We've already talked about how sunscreens can help prevent wrinkles; moisturizers do, too. It prevents them, not eliminates them. If you are going to try a product which contains an alpha-hydroxy acid, I recommend that it be a moisturizer. You'll use it every day (you have to or the AHAs won't work).

When buying, go for the lower-priced brands. There is not one iota of difference between them and the outrageously priced ones.

Limit Your Supplies

I used to buy every bottle and jar of moisturizers, toners, masks, you name it. If it came in a cute bottle or made outrageous claims, I bought it. I never really used the stuff I bought either. I just threw it in the closet. I used to think that a new product would give me a little lift, but it never really did. It just made me feel bad for spending all that money. I have lots more control now and try really hard to stick to my tried and true products. It's smarter to put your time and money into investigating the products that do work. Once you find them, stick with them. *

Buy according to your skin type and how the moisturizer feels. Be very careful about added fragrances, particularly botanicals. "Natural" fragrances and products have proliferated in the past few years and the advertising for them makes it seem as though you were doing something virtuous by using them. You're not, but you may irritate your skin. Try to use a fragrance-free product; your perfume should be all the fragrance you need.

Toners

Toners and astringents are meant to remove oil and in some cases minimize the size of large pores on the face. The difference between them is that astringents usually contain alcohol, which is very drying, and toners don't (witch hazel is often the active ingredient). Alcohol is beneficial to unclog pores after a good sweaty workout (use a moisturizer after to rehydrate skin), but can be too drying for normal use.

Those with acne or blemishes can benefit from toners to dry those areas. None of us really need these products, but they do leave skin feeling fresh and tingly. Used sparingly they won't damage skin.

To apply, pour a small amount on a clean cotton ball. Wipe skin until cotton balls (use a few) come away clean.

Masks

Masks are an every-once-in-a-while beauty treat. You don't *really* need to use a mask, but they sure feel good. Masks work to exfoliate dead cells and deep-clean pores (not as thoroughly as a facial though), to give skin a smoother texture and a healthy glow. The products come in gels, creams, and a claylike form. There are wash-off and peel-off products. Which ones you use depends on your skin type and preference. Read package labels to determine which is best for your skin type. Generally, clay-based masks are best for oily skin, while creams are good for dry skin (those with built-in moisturizers are even better).

If you have oily skin, you can use a mask about every two weeks (this won't damage skin, but it seems a little excessive). Those with dry skin should limit masks to once a month. If you have combination skin, you can apply the mask only to oily areas.

Facials

The ultimate skin-pampering treat is a deep-cleansing facial in a salon. Facials clean skin and, if done well, leave you feeling relaxed. A good facial takes about an hour and includes: an evaluation of your skin type and condition (here's where you ask what type of skin you have!); a deep cleaning; massage and moisturizing; and then a gentle steaming to open pores. The esthetician (that's what facial providers are called) will then gently squeeze blackheads (they call it unclogging pores, but I know what they're doing) and apply a toner. They will then usually apply a mask, which stays on for about ten minutes. After the mask is removed and skin is cleaned one last time, the esthetician will rub in a moisturizer, and if you're really lucky, she'll give you a neck and shoulder massage.

Now, be prepared—the first couple of times I got facials I ended up with red, blotchy skin that proceeded to break out over the next few days. A deep-cleansing facial is an all-out assault on your skin. If you have problems following a facial, call the salon and ask what to do. Next time you have a facial, explain what happened. The esthetician will be gentler and use less irritating products.

Pimples, Blackheads, and Blotches

It never fails. You have a big party to go to tonight and you wake up with a hunker of a zit right in the middle of your nose. What's going on? Didn't we already go through this as teenagers? It seems so unfair to get acne as an adult, doesn't it? Well, we all get pimples, even me. Adult acne is not like kid acne. We usually get one or two pimples at a time, usually at the same time of month. It's caused by all sorts of things: hormonal changes, heredity, stress, pregnancy, irritating skin-care products, the position of the moon (just kidding). But really, it's hard to know why we get that giant pimple at that special moment. You can do the best you can to avoid acne by washing and caring for skin, but chances are you are going to get the occasional breakout anyway.

What to do when a pimple rears it's ugly head? Don't squeeze it no matter how much you want to. Squeezing can force the inflammation deeper into skin and cause infection and a nasty scar. There are a couple of things you can try for quick relief:

* Dab a bit of benzoyl peroxide on a cotton swab and apply directly to pimple. Benzoyl peroxide is found in almost all over-the-counter acne medications—check labels.

* Dab a bit of lemon juice onto the pimple to help dry it out.

* See your dermatologist. Dermatologists can inject blemishes with cortisone (it takes two minutes and the pimple will almost disappear by the next day). If the pimple is infected, they may also give you oral antibiotics, which work in a day or two.

If you have pitted skin from acne scars, there are many new treatments available that are less invasive than dermabrasion (this sounds truly disgusting), which is a deep scrubbing of skin done under general anesthesia. Here's a breakdown of what's available:

My Savior

I never like to push products on anyone because I know people have to find the best ones for them, but I have to mention the one thing I am never without: Acnomel (you can buy it in any drugstore). Great name, huh? I can't live without it. It is my miracle pimple cure. If I even feel a pimple coming on I apply a dab of Acnomel before bed and by morning the pimple has dried up and calmed down. I have a tube in every bathroom, at work and in my travel makeup kit. If they ever stop making it, I'd have to buy enough to last forever. I love this stuff! *

Superficial Facial Peels

This kind of light peel is great for getting blemishes under control. It sort of lets you start over with a clean palette. A diluted glycolic acid solution is applied to face for about five to ten minutes, depending on severity of blemishes. It is then washed off. There will be a mild redness for a week or so, but little or no pain. You can have a few in a row (every month) to really wipe out blemishes without submitting to a deeper dermabrasion. Cost is about $100 per treatment.

Collagen Injections

The good part about collagen injections is that they are quick and almost painless, with no down time. The bad part is that you have to have them redone every so often because the collagen is absorbed into the body. The other drawback is the cost ($300 to $400 per visit). This procedure is best to fill only a handful of deep scars, not for the whole face.

Fat Injections

Fat injections last a little longer than collagen injections, but they have to get the fat from somewhere. They get it from you by harvesting it (yuck!) from a fatty area in your body, usually the stomach. The procedure is done under local anesthesia (which means you're awake) and does cause some redness and swelling. About 30 percent of the fat will stay put, the rest is reabsorbed in body. If you have the procedure repeated, more of the fat will stay there the next time. The cost is about $1,500.

Laser Resurfacing

Laser surgery is here to stay, but right now there are a lot of overzealous doctors out there firing away without the necessary training. A misfired laser can result in a worse scar, so be sure your doctor is qualified to use one. Lasers work very well to remove red or raised scars, and do remove most acne scars. The effects of resurfacing last about three years (maybe more, it hasn't been studied yet), and your skin will be red and sore for a few weeks. Full results appear after three months. Cost is about $2,000 for specific areas; more for a full face resurfacing.

Beware of Gimmicks

Shortly after I moved to New York to be with Frank, I was getting my nails done in a salon when I overheard a woman talking about getting her face waxed. *Wow,* I thought, *I've always been so hairy on my face, maybe this is the magic solution!* I asked this woman about it, and she said it was great and only cost $100. I signed right up. This was one of the biggest mistakes I ever made. There was a reason I'd never heard of facial waxing before: It's very damaging to skin and most salons would never recommend it. I was broken out for months. All my pores were clogged and I had the biggest pimples you've ever seen. I was better off with the hair. I learned that you really have to look into treatments before you leap right in. If you've never heard of it before there's probably a good reason. ✳

Hair Removal

Part of caring for your skin is removing unwanted hair from legs, underarms, bikini line, and if you're dark, from your lip and chin. There are a number of ways to remove hair, almost all of which you can do at home. Electrolysis is really the only procedure that needs to be done in a salon by a professional. Here are the pros and cons of the different methods:

SHAVING

PROS:
• Works for all areas except lip and chin.
• It's cheap, pain-free (if you're careful), and removes both coarse and thin hair.

CONS:
• Hair regrows quickly.

TWEEZING

PROS:
• Best for eyebrows, or other facial hair.
• It's cheap and you can control contours and shapes.

CONS:
• It hurts. Regrowth occurs in about a week.

WAXING

PROS:
• Good for all areas except face. Best for legs and bikini line.
• If done at home, can cost about $5 per application.
• Lasts about two to four weeks, depending on your rate of regrowth.

CONS:
• It hurts.
• You have to let hair grow out to at least a quarter of an inch for waxing to work.
• Salon costs are about $10 for bikini line, can be up to $60 for full leg and bikini line.

DEPILATORIES

PROS:
• Good for body and face.
• These are chemicals that remove hair more thoroughly than a shaver.
• They are cheap (about $4) and last about a week.

CONS:
• Requires waiting with smelly chemicals all over you.
• Can irritate skin.

BLEACHING

PROS:
• Can be done at home and used on arms and face.
• Cheap (about $4 a kit), quick, and lasts about two weeks.

CONS:
• Can burn skin, cause breakouts or redness.

ELECTROLYSIS

PROS:
• Permanently removes hair.
• Is best for small areas like lip and chin, or stray hairs on breasts or stomach.

CONS:
• Very expensive (about $40 per hour) and time-consuming (even a small area can take many appointments to get rid of all hairs).

Part IV

Self-Image

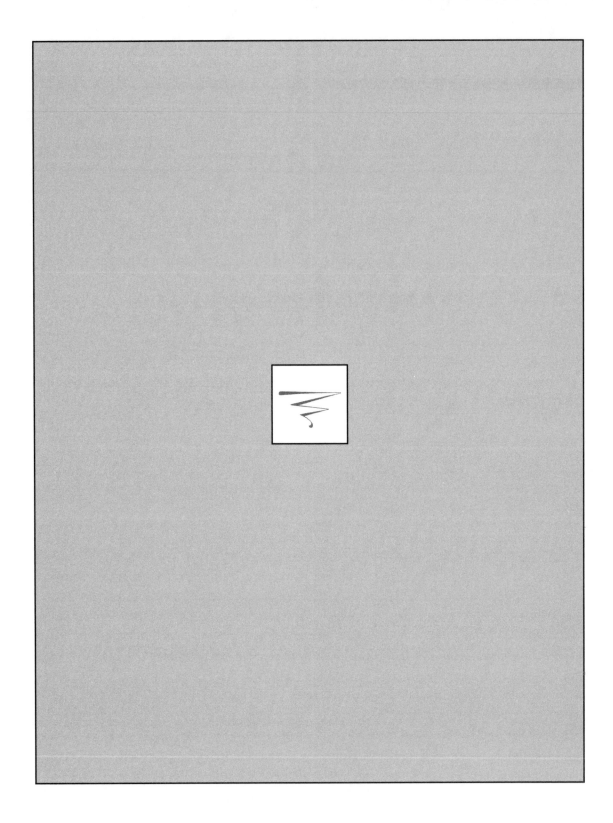

Chapter 14

Magazines,
the Media, and You

Fashion magazines have always held an attraction for us. We started reading them as teenagers with *Seventeen,* then moved on to *Mademoiselle,* and then to *Vogue* and *Harper's Bazaar.* We even went through that period when we bought *Cosmo* to learn to be sexy. We read magazines with the excitement of things that were to come in our lives. I know I hoped I might someday look like the girls in the magazines, didn't you? That was the point, right? But I didn't look like them, and I didn't know why. I know it made me feel like I wasn't good enough. The little voice in my head said, *Your life would be so perfect if only you were different. What's wrong with you? Why don't you look like the models in all of the fashion magazines?*

I know now that I *can* look that way. We all can. But what would we have to give up for it? I know because I eventually was one of those girls. I did become a model. I paid a big price; I threw up every day. Even though I was working steadily, I felt like I couldn't hold on to it. It's like borrowing a great outfit from a friend that fits perfectly, having your hair and makeup done, and for that one moment looking better than you've ever looked before. Like Cinderella you go to the ball and have a wonderful time. Then you come back home, take off the dress, and get into your jammies and you're just you. You know you'll never look that great again. That's how

I felt all the time. *Okay, I pulled it off today, but what about tomorrow?* It was such a struggle. That's what makes me the saddest, that awful struggle we have with our looks. Even though I was a model I never *felt* like the other models looked. They made it look so easy. It wasn't easy for me. I was willing to make myself sick just so that I would not be me. Or just so that I would be me but thinner.

Boy, was that stupid. Of course I want to be me, and my size is just a part of who I am. But we always want what we don't have, don't we? If only I were thinner, we say. Or blonder. Or taller. Or whatever we aren't. I know that models give up a lot to have it all. They eat tofu and lettuce, and drink hot water with lemon. (Do you want to eat that way? I don't.) Do you want to work out every day? I certainly don't. Even if I wanted to work out every day, I just don't have the time. It's worth it to models because they are highly paid and admired for their looks—it's their job—but you aren't and shouldn't judge yourself by these false images you see in magazines and ads.

Reality Check

Now that doesn't mean you can cheer and say, "Hey, Linda says it's okay for me to be fat and unhealthy. Yippee!" You *should* read fashion magazines to inspire yourself to make changes. We all look better when we're the weight we should be. I don't care who you are; weight makes a difference. It doesn't mean that you can't look pretty unless you are tall and thin and have perfect hair. That's not what it's about. It's about liking yourself and doing what you can to like yourself even more. I like who I am now, but it took a long time to get here. I used to let other people and images define the standards that I tried to live up to but could never meet. Now that I'm older and a little bit more secure about what I've accomplished (bumpy thighs and all), it makes me so crazy to think that other women struggle with this same sort of media condemnation of their looks.

I read the fashion magazines and see television coverage of the big fashion shows and it defeats me. Am I so old that I don't understand the clothes? It can't *just* be me. The clothes are designed and photographed for young, thin things. You might fit that category right now, but we all fall out of that loop eventually. We know we can't wear a sleeveless formfitting dress forever, yet we still feel intimidated by fashion magazines because that's what they say we should wear. And sometimes you do wear something you see in a magazine even though it's totally inappropriate—age and size—for who you are now. You cave in because you don't have the confidence to choose the styles you know you should wear—styles that look and feel good on *you.*

Who Are They Selling to?

We look and read and feel awful about ourselves because we don't look like the "experts" say we are supposed to. I mean, I opened a fashion magazine a few days ago and saw a pencil-thin model wearing lime-green capri pants with a pink see-through top flying open to the navel. You will *never*, in a million years, catch me wearing anything that gives the world an up-close and personal view of my stomach and arms. It's not because I think I'm fat; it's about age and what's appropriate for me. I would look ridiculous. Like a grown woman trying to look like a teenager. You probably wouldn't wear a shirt like that, either. How could you? *Where* would you? And why should you? Just because some designer convinced a New York fashion editor to take a picture of one of his outfits? I don't think so.

I wouldn't mind if one or two stories in each issue showed clothes like this, but often the entire editorial package for the month is about the same kind of look. I want a magazine that can do fashion across the board; styles that range from those for a twenty-year-old to those for a fifty-year-old. I want models that look my age. That doesn't mean I'm over-the-hill and can't dress well. But I want models that have my attitude: *I can look great at fifty. I can wear stylish clothes. I am sexy.* That's what I want to see. I want to see clothes that are more suitable for most women's lifestyles and budgets. I want to see models who look more like us. Don't you?

So why do we see models wearing ridiculous clothes in impossibly small sizes on magazine pages? Well, the fact is magazines are driven by advertisers. That's where they make their money and that's where a good part of their attention is focused. Of course, the companies that buy advertising want to see their products displayed and given a sort of editorial stamp of approval. If the editors choose these styles, they must be the best, right? Sometimes that is true. Sometimes there is a trade-off: ad space for editorial coverage. Of course, editors will never

Seeing Is *Not* Believing

I once took a client shopping. I can't tell you her name because she'd kill me. D.L. saw a three-piece silk suit in a fashion magazine. It was a silky, unconstructed number in an orange, melony kind of color. We found the suit in a store and she tried it on. It looked awful. It hung horribly on her—talk about unconstructed! The skirt was also way too long and she looked dumpy.

D.L. couldn't understand it. When she looked in the mirror all she saw was the magazine page. She was going to buy that suit—over my dead body. I know, and now you will, too, that the way clothes are styled in magazines are rarely the way you will find them in stores. First of all, stylists use clothespins in the back for a couturelike fit. Sample skirts are often made shorter than the ones sold for mass consumption. Studio lighting may even slightly affect the color you see. The point here is that you have to try hard to buy only clothes that look good on *you*, not the ones that you think you should buy because they looked terrific on a model. ✳

admit that they show certain styles just because a company buys advertising, but it plays more than a subliminal role in their selections.

Okay, so still, why do magazines have to show those clothes on super-skinny gorgeous girls who are ten years younger than their core audience? Six feet tall, size six, perfect hair, etc. The girls we love to hate, yet want to be. This is where no one will really take responsibility. The fashion editors say that the designers only provide sample clothes in small sizes, so they have to hire thin models to wear them. The designers say that modeling agencies only take on girls who are small, so they have to make samples to fit them, otherwise their clothes won't be used. The modeling agencies say that magazines and designers would never hire a bigger model because— surprise!—they won't fit the clothes. The fact is that most clothes do look better on a tall, thin woman, and of course, designers want to sell their clothes, so it's a vicious cycle. And it probably isn't going to change. So you and I have to learn how to deal with these images and not let them make us feel bad about ourselves.

I am not saying that fashion magazines are all bad. I read them. I get ideas from them. What I am saying is that you shouldn't believe that you're not good enough just because you're not sixteen, and tall, thin, and perfectly muscled. You're you and we're working on building *your* confidence.

Early Damage

Little girls hear early on that looks matter, and believe it or not, they are affected by it very much. My manager, Jonathan Pillot, and his wife, writer Shawne Cooper, have a five-year-old daughter named Maia. Maia came home from school one day, looked in the refrigerator, and pulled out a snack. "Does this have fat in it?" she said. Shawne thought that was a strange question coming from a kindergartner and asked her why she wanted to know that. Well, it turns out that the mother of another girl in her class has been telling her daughter that she is fat and must only eat low-fat foods. According to Shawne, this girl is not fat, but the mother is pencil-thin and obviously cares that her daughter be as well. We all have to be careful about what we say concerning weight to young girls; our words affect them more than we think. Do we really want five-year-olds obsessing about fat? I think if we made a big deal out of their abilities, rather than their looks, we'd help grow healthier women. Let's all stop talking about fat, and especially judging women by it. It really is what's inside that counts. ✳

Why Looks Matter

The development of our self-image started when we were young girls and first began to realize that looks matter. We were too young to understand that all the media images that show who we are supposed to be are false. All we saw was that the pretty girls got the boys and more attention from teachers and other adults. Not just magazines, but the world was telling us that looks matter. And they do. I wish they didn't, but they do. It's important to look pulled-together and pretty. People respond to it. We respond to it. We like the way it feels. But what we have to remember is that pretty is not just one look, no matter what you see in magazines. Every one of us defines pretty in a different way when we are *really* being honest with ourselves. We know that we are not all the same, yet other people still find something attractive about each one of us. *You* have to believe you're attractive, or that you can be. Growing up I never felt that I was pretty, and yet I have had a successful career in an industry where looks matter in a serious way. Frank has always said that I am a pretty girl with an ugly girl's personality. Since I never *really* believed I was pretty, I worked hard to develop a personality that people would be attracted to. Of course, I *was* being hired for my looks, but I thought it was my humor and talent that people loved. Not only have I had this great career, I have been married three times. Actually I'm very embarrassed about that, but the point is that three men fell head-over-heels in love with me—at least that's what they told me—and thought I was attractive. Now you might think I'm pretty, too. You might say, "What is she talking about?" You see, it's how I feel about myself that matters. All of this happened to me and still, I thought I was unattractive. It's taken years of having it pounded into my head, but yes, I now believe my looks are okay.

Fighting Back

If I had it my way, I would supply each parent of a newborn girl with a copy of *Reviving Ophelia* by Mary Pipher, Ph.D. At the hospital, parents should get a package of diapers and this book. It's about saving the selves of adolescent girls. The author has done mounds of research and treated hundreds of girls in the area of self-image. She talks about all the confusing messages young girls receive about their looks and abilities, and she gives us instructions on how to get through the maze. I read this book and cried. It described me in so many ways. Although I cried, it was a great help on the path to understanding why I did all the crazy things I did—like bulimia. It also made me mad. I didn't have to be that way. You and I are adults now and can fend off the bad feelings about not being perfect, but wouldn't it be great if we could prevent the next generation from *ever* having to feel that way?

Self-image and fashion are intrinsically tied together. How we look absolutely affects how we feel. I know I can't let designers and fashion editors and movie directors tell me how I should look anymore. I have to feel good about me. A lot of women feel this way and I believe that we are finally getting the message across. Fashion as we have known it is growing extinct. There are fewer rules. Nobody is going to tell me what skirt length I can wear. I know what length looks good on me, and that's what I am going to wear. You should, too. Whatever it is. Length. Color.

Fabric. You do know what looks best on you, or at least you will after you read this book. If you have dimpled thighs, like me, you should *never* wear a miniskirt, even if you see them in every magazine and store. If you can't find a skirt that's right for you, you have options: Have one made or wait until the style you want comes around again; it will. Don't ever buy just to meet somebody else's standard of fashion.

Looking at magazines, watching fashion shows, going to stores, reading this book, are all ways you learn about fashion and how you can look the best you know how. They are tools for you to use; you are not supposed to follow their instructions exactly. If we all did, we'd all look the same. You're not supposed to look like me. The key is to learn how to take what you need and leave the rest.

The rest of the world's attention to weight is no longer important to me. If TV shows and magazines and movies want to show teeny-tiny women as the ideal, let them. It's my feelings about my weight and how I look that are important. And I do care about my weight. I want to be healthy. I want to fit into the thousands of dollars of clothes in my closet and, mostly, I just don't want to obsess over whether other people think I'm too fat. You'll see how I have come to terms with all these demons in the next chapter.

Chapter 15

Weight, Yuck

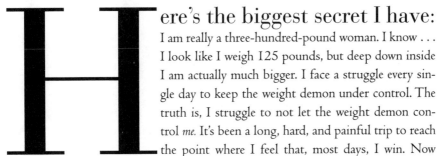ere's the biggest secret I have: I am really a three-hundred-pound woman. I know . . . I look like I weigh 125 pounds, but deep down inside I am actually much bigger. I face a struggle every single day to keep the weight demon under control. The truth is, I struggle to not let the weight demon control *me*. It's been a long, hard, and painful trip to reach the point where I feel that, most days, I win. Now understand, I don't always win. In fact, in my life I have gone for long periods when I didn't win. Bulimia was my constant companion for twenty-five years. I only stopped because I knew it would kill me. Where does that powerful voice come from (*Come on, little girl, just one doughnut . . .*) that makes us do such crazy things? I had a secret life that no one knew about, yet it was my *whole* life.

I don't think I will ever reach the place I really want to be, which is to not care, or ever even think about my obsession with food. What a wonderful day that would be! Can you imagine what it would be like to wake up and eat whatever you wanted, all day long, and never once consider the effect on your waistline? Believe it or not, I'm kind of like that now. I don't eat the amount of food I used to, but I've reached the point where I don't have to deprive myself. Right here we'll talk about the strategies for coping with the weight demon. So let's sit down with some popcorn (no butter, please), and we'll go over all of it. Don't think for a minute that I'm not just like you. I have to hear it every day, so this will be good for both of us.

It's actually hard to write about this. Weight. All that it means. What it represents. How it affects, changes, influences, tricks, defines, intimidates, belittles, depresses, controls, and dictates me. I have so many feelings about weight, and I don't want to leave out one detail. It's almost as though if I tell you my story completely, honestly, it will somehow make the whole problem easier to handle . . . for you and for me.

It seems like I have been thinking about my weight my whole life. I guess I have—it's certainly been a part of each day for as long as I can remember. Should I or shouldn't I hate myself today? Fighting to stay "good" just another day. I was like a runaway train. Why was I like this, I thought? I was always a little out of control. Finally I discovered bulimia—fabulous—a way to eat everything, anything I wanted and no one would know. I was finally in control of something: eating and then purging. I could eat a dozen doughnuts (and I did), a quart of milk and then throw it all up. I stayed thin. It was great! Or so I thought. I didn't realize at the time that I was doing permanent damage to my body, especially my teeth. All I cared about was being thin.

So what are we really talking about here? I overate for all the reasons we all overeat: as a substitute for confronting problems. My eating was out of control because I was out of control. I always wanted to be someone else. If I felt trapped or frustrated or afraid, if I felt unattractive, old, unappreciated, I went to food. My friend, my comfort place. I even went to food when I was happy. I even ate when I was sick. Can you believe that!

If I'm not eating, I'm thinking about eating. This is a problem I have always lived with. So what has changed? Have I changed? Yes and no. Are you surprised I say "no"? Let me explain.

I should first simply say to you that I don't really know what this is all about. Why I have a problem with food and someone else doesn't. I have never known the cause but I keep searching for the truth to free myself, to put this all-consuming topic to rest. I am so much better now than ever before so maybe I am finally on the right road. Here's what Linda Dano does now—most of the time.

First, let's understand that food addiction, eating disorders like bulimia and anorexia, are all *real* problems. And unlike alcohol or drugs, food is something you can't just walk away from. You have to eat. So, right off the bat you have to learn to deal with it. Food is here to stay. That's why I think it is the most difficult of addictions to beat. Food is in your face every single day!

I am trembling a little as I write this. I feel like I should say something funny or clever. But you and I know that there is nothing funny about this. Sure we can make jokes about it, but inside it's not funny. The pain we feel when we are overweight or struggling not to eat too much goes deep, deep down to our very core. We know how bad this feels, don't we? But we really can change the way we feel about food and ourselves. If you think you can do it yourself, I'm here to tell you you can't. I thought I could. I thought that if I tried really hard, I could control myself. All that did was to make me think about food more. And hate myself more when I failed. I finally had to get help from someone who taught me a different way to eat and live. It's the hardest thing I've ever done. I did it; you can, too.

It all started in 1994. I got on the scale one day, and I was shocked to see that I weighed 170 pounds. Since I usually weighed between 115 and 125, this was a substantial weight gain. How did this happen? Not only was my health on the line, but maybe my job, my whole career was, too. I was scared. Really scared. This was the biggest I'd ever been. How was I going to lose this weight? Could I lose this weight? It was so much to lose. What if I couldn't do it? It depressed me to think about dieting yet again. Dieting made me so conscious of my weight. It was on my mind all the time. Was I a good girl today or a bad girl? It was so awful.

One day, out of the blue, I got a call from a company that wanted me to do an infomercial and lend my name to its weight-loss program. I immediately said no. One, because I just don't do infomercials and, two, because I'd been on enough diets to know that nothing really works. I wasn't going to try to sell a diet that was going to cost people a lot of money and still make them miserable. The doctor who developed the program, Nancy Bonios, Ph.D., said she was going to send me the information about her program anyway. It consisted of eight audiotapes, a videotape, a guide, and a personal workbook.

I popped one of the tapes into the cassette player of my car during a drive to our house in Connecticut. I was fascinated by what I was hearing. It had to do with my mind, not my body. It had to do with controlling what I was going to eat and that it was my choice that determined how much and what I should eat. All of a sudden, the deprivation I had experienced with dieting was gone. This program actually freed me from my dependency on food. I was going to be the one in control!

I can't tell you everything about The Bonios Plan™ because all of the material would fill a separate book. Fortunately, the publisher of the plan, the Chatham Institute™, has allowed me to share the basic principles with you. (I am not trying to sell you the plan, but if you want to learn more, you can call Chatham Institute's toll-free helpline at 800–760–5490.)

Basic Principles of
The Bonios Plan™

Principle #1. Only Eat When
Physically Hungry

First, eat only when you are physically hungry, which you do by reinterpreting your hunger signals. This principle will help you reestablish natural eating habits and reduce your food intake to the level your body actually needs.

TOOL #1. MAKE PEACE WITH THE IDEA OF HUNGER

Hunger is not a dangerous condition that must be avoided through continuous eating and snacking. It is a natural state, and your body will signal you that your stomach is empty and ready to receive more food. By permitting yourself to feel the true sensation of hunger, you will learn to eat only when you feel the need to refuel.

TOOL #2. REDEFINE HUNGER

A growling stomach is often not an empty stomach. True hunger means your stomach is empty, and it is time to think about what you would enjoy eating.

TOOL #3. REMEMBER YOUR STOMACH CLOCK

Food stays in your stomach for six to nine hours, which you probably know if you have ever had a general anesthetic. Your doctor would have asked you not to eat for at least eight hours before the procedure to ensure that your stomach empties first. Most of us forget how long food stays in our stomach, and we're surprised when we realize that we are not feeling true physical hunger.

TOOL #4. GET OFF AUTOMATIC

The clock does not signal true physical hunger, your stomach does. So stop eating by the clock or by other external signals. Before you eat, ask yourself (a) when was the last time I ate, and (b) could I still have food in my stomach? If yes, then don't eat.

Instead, drink something. Many times you are not really hungry, but thirsty. Or chew gum. This will satisfy the natural urge to chew something, or feel something in your mouth. Finally, write down your feelings. Expressing yourself on paper when you are in a bingeing mood will often stop the sensation, and may help you identify your real reasons for eating. This will satisfy the need to deal with your emotions, instead of covering them up or pushing them down with food.

Principle #2. Stop Eating When Hunger Disappears

By stopping when hunger disappears, we no longer eat beyond our stomach's real capacity. This principle helps us learn to stop eating when we have eaten a fist-sized portion, and eliminate all of the unnecessary extra fuel that our body stores as fat. We learn how to stop eating by "Legalizing All Food" and by "Eating Properly.".

TOOL #1. "LEGALIZE ALL FOOD"—YOU CAN'T GET ENOUGH OF WHAT YOU DON'T REALLY WANT

Depriving yourself of the foods you *really* want will simply increase the craving, and can lead to binging or compulsive overeating. Deprivation is part of the unhealthy diet cycle, and fake foods and substitutes aren't fooling anybody, including your body. Don't eat an apple if you really want chocolate cake.

TOOL #2. "LEGALIZE ALL FOOD"—IT'S ONLY FUEL

Food is nothing more than fuel for your body. By breaking out of the diet mentality, we discard the old obsessions about "good" and "bad" foods, along with the "shoulds" about eating. Food is not dangerous or illegal—it is *simply fuel.*

TOOL #3. "LEGALIZE ALL FOOD"—EAT EXACTLY WHAT YOU WANT

When you are physically hungry, you will eat only what you are in the mood for. Eating what tastes best will put you in control of your food choices, and enable you to respond to your body's natural signals for different food needs. You will satisfy your hunger, stop your craving, get the fuel your body needs—and find it much easier to *stop* eating.

TOOL #4. "EATING PROPERLY"—FIST IN YOUR LAP

Your stomach is about the size of your fist. By holding your fist in your lap while you eat, you will be able to gauge the amount of food you can consume at each meal. Eating beyond this natural capacity will make you uncomfortable—and overweight.

TOOL #5. "EATING PROPERLY"—DIVIDE YOUR PLATE IN HALF

Mentally or physically divide the food on your plate in half. Of course you can eat the second half—it is your food—but only after you have eaten the first half, slowly savoring each bite, and find that if, after pausing fifteen minutes, you are still physically hungry.

TOOL #6. "EATING PROPERLY"—EAT SLOWLY AND SAVOR EACH BITE

By taking small bites and eating slowly, you will better be able to tell when your stomach is filled to its natural capacity. By slowing down, you will enjoy your favorite foods even more, so make a point of intentionally savoring each and every bite.

TOOL #7. "EATING PROPERLY"—LOOK FOR THE "SIGH"

When you feel the urge to "sigh" or take a deep breath, your stomach is telling you it is full. It is time to stop eating so that you do not overeat and feel uncomfortable. No matter how delicious or expensive the food is, it's just fuel.

TOOL #8. "EATING PROPERLY"—NEVER EAT PAST FULL

When you have filled your stomach to its natural capacity, stop eating. It is okay to throw food away or save it for later—just don't store leftovers in your stomach. There is never a good reason to overeat. Since our tendency is to eat what is in front of us, push your plate off to the side when you stop eating.

Principle #3. Change Your Thinking and Habits from "Fat" to "Thin"

You cannot become permanently thin if you are thinking and acting like a fat person. Studies in mind/body medicine have demonstrated the powerful interplay between your thoughts and your body, so it is important to cancel negative thoughts and replace them with positive new thoughts. This we do through Cancel and Replace tools, Metabolism Suggestions, and Guided Imagery.

TOOL #1. CANCEL AND REPLACE

Stress causes a variety of negative health effects, including the release of insulin, which turns nutrients to fat. Listen to your internal thoughts and self-talk. Cancel all negative "fat" thoughts and images, and replace them with loving and positive ones. Relax around food, and stop thinking of food as fattening. Instead, tell yourself all food now makes you healthy and thin.

Weighing yourself is stressful, and can sabotage your progress. Since naturally thin people do not need scales in their lives, stop using yours. You can measure your success by your loose clothes and new behavior.

TOOL #2. METABOLISM SUGGESTIONS

Your thoughts and feelings trigger constant changes and responses in your body. You can use this powerful mind/body connection to create positive changes through "metabolism suggestions." Choose and repeat a phrase describing how food will react in your body, such as: "Everything I eat causes me to lose weight, and I am becoming thinner and more attractive now," or "My metabolism is speeding up, making me thinner and thinner now." Remember, you don't have to believe these positive affirmations are completely true when you begin, but the more you repeat them, the more they will come true.

TOOL #3. GUIDED IMAGERY

The image you have of yourself influences your thoughts and actions, so changing your image from fat to thin is important. Professional athletes use this powerful technique to visualize themselves as they want to be, and you can too. By creating a thin and attractive image of yourself in your mind's eye, you will accelerate your progress toward achieving it.

It may help to use the following statement as a reminder when you eat: *Every time I eat I always eat properly. I only eat exactly what I want. I take small bites. I chew slowly and thoroughly, savoring the flavor. I pause between bites and check with my stomach to sense its hunger level. I notice I become full and satisfied after eating a small amount of food. As soon as I notice this, I happily stop eating. I push my plate away with food still on it, feeling proud to do so. As a result, I'm getting thinner every day.*

The Changes I've Made

The Bonios Plan™ hit me like a smack in the face. Like a wake-up call. I never need to go on a crazy diet again because I can now eat whatever I want. I initially lost thirty-five pounds in three months using the Bonios philosophy. Sure, I may gain five pounds or so every now and then (and hate myself when I do), but most of the time I can eat properly and be happy about it.

I still cook gourmet meals for Frank and my mother, I just don't eat everything on my plate. I used to have to make detours around doughnut stores because I knew if I came close I would have to run and eat a few—or a dozen. Now I drive or walk right by. If I feel like going in, I do. I may only eat half a doughnut and throw the rest away, but I don't deprive myself or feel on ounce of guilt. That's the biggest change I've made. I don't have to obsess over food anymore because I know that I can eat whatever I want whenever I'm hungry, and still stay thin.

I will never be totally over my problems with food. I know that. But now it is not such a huge part of my life. This release has freed me to enjoy other parts of life. I feel like a new person. I am a new person. You can be a new, thin person, too. If you want to be. Just don't let being fat make you feel like a bad person. It doesn't have anything to do with who you *really* are.

Chapter 16

Medical Miracles . . .
and More

Ihave never had plastic surgery, but I can't
guarantee that I won't. Ask me Tuesday at 3:00 and I'll say, *Oh, yes, I need
a face-lift.* Ask me Wednesday at 2:00 and I might say, *Nah, I changed my
mind.* Will I, won't I, will I . . . oh, I don't know. As a matter of fact, I
probably will someday. I have had dental implants, which I guess can be
considered a form of cosmetic surgery. Believe me, it *felt* like surgery. I
had some teeth that were beyond repair (bulimia caused) and the alternative would have been to lose even more teeth and have a bridge made.
I had to do something; I couldn't possibly have shown up at work one day and said,
"Sorry, guys, Felicia isn't going to have teeth from now on." The procedure, which
takes about six months in total, was painful and inconvenient. But the results are
incredible. I feel so much better about myself. I can smile with confidence and that
has made a huge difference in how I present myself.

My experience with my teeth leads me to believe that I would get the same
feeling from an eye-lift, or even a full face-lift if I needed one. I am not worried
about looking old—although in my business, I should be—I'm more worried about
not feeling good about myself, because I've been there before. But before I have any
surgery, I would want to know what all of my options are and how to go about finding a good plastic surgeon. No, not good, great. One thing that makes me think

twice about plastic surgery is the fear that something would go wrong. What if the surgeon is having a bad day? What if I look like his ex-wife? What if he is coming down with the flu? What if he really wanted to be a fashion designer? Okay, so I'm a little paranoid, but it *could* happen. And what if I don't heal right? It's so scary, isn't it? Even though I am investigating all of this information for *you*, it's really for us. Let's take notes and file them away until the day we need them. If we need them. If we want them . . . if, if, if . . .

Why Do You Want Surgery?

This is a question you have to answer before you even head to a doctor's office. If you want to make surgical changes to your face and/or body because the way you look is making you feel bad about yourself or is holding you back (you never go swimming because you can't stand your saddlebag thighs), then by all means go for it. But if you think surgery is going to change your life, you need to think again. (If you don't look like Cindy Crawford now, you won't after surgery either.) Bigger breasts aren't going to save a failing marriage and a face-lift won't necessarily help you land a promotion at work. Make sure you are doing this for you.

How Do You Find a Surgeon?

As I said, I wouldn't want just a surgeon, I'd want the best—for me and for you. You find a qualified surgeon by doing a little checking and relying on your own instincts. Any licensed doctors can perform cosmetic surgery if they want to and a patient will let them. Cosmetic surgery is not a specialty that has its own board certification. The official title of the doctor who is *qualified* to perform cosmetic surgery is plastic and reconstructive surgeon. Other doctors who are trained to do cosmetic surgery are ENTs (otorhinolaryngologists—ear, nose, and throat doctors), who perform facial surgeries, and eye doctors (ophthalmologic surgeons), who often perform cosmetic eye surgery. All three of these specialties have boards that oversee the training and testing of doctors. You absolutely want a surgeon who is board-certified. This guarantees the highest level of training available.

Do not be swayed by a wall full of framed certificates that look important but may not mean much. Doctors belong to tons of organizations that have nothing to do with medicine. An official-sounding name such as American Academy of

Professional Doctors may just be a group of doctors who like to fly-fish together. The only certificates that mean anything to you are the doctor's medical degree, board certification, and two professional organizations: the American Society of Plastic and Reconstructive Surgeons (ASPRS) and the American Academy of Facial and Reconstructive Surgery. All members of the ASPRS are board-certified and must be nominated to join by their peers. To find out if a surgeon you are considering is board-certified, call ASPRS at 800–635–0635. Members of the American Academy of Facial and Reconstructive Surgery are also board-certified and specialize in facial surgery. (To find members or check credentials call 800–333–3223. If you don't have a surgeon in mind, both organizations will provide you with a list of board-certified surgeons in your area.)

Your surgeon should also have hospital privileges at a local hospital. Privileges allow the doctor to admit and treat patients in the hospital. If you require hospitalization after surgery you will be assured that your own doctor can treat you. Also, hospitals are picky about who they let work in their facilities, so it's another level of protection for you.

There are a couple of other places to look if you do not have a particular surgeon in mind: A book called *The Directory of Medical Specialists* (available in most libraries) lists every board-certified doctor in the United States. Your county medical society will also have a list of local doctors. You should also ask your family doctor or gynecologist for recommendations. The medical community is very small and most good doctors know who the other good ones are.

Finally, use your own judgment. Make an appointment for a consultation to discuss the procedure you want done. The doctor should spend as much time with you as you need and answer all of your questions, even the stupid ones. You need to feel comfortable with this person so don't be intimidated. Ask all the questions you can think of.

What to Watch Out for

There are a couple of clues to look for that may tell you that the surgeon is thinking more about gaining another patient than giving you the results you want. These are not absolutes, but rather things you should question:

✳ You go in for a face-lift and the surgeon suggests you also need a nose job and breast lift to look "perfect." You think you need a little pick-me-up and now you feel like a horror show. This doctor is going too far, and you should ask him why he recommends these procedures and how they will affect your appearance. *You* decide what you want, not the surgeon.

✴ The doctor shows you before-and-after photos of other patients. What do you care what other patients look like? The surgeon should use medical photos to describe the procedure that you want and tell you what results *you* can expect.

✴ The surgeon promises results that sound too good to be true. They may be. Ask why your surgery will be so successful. It's possible that what you want done will truly improve your looks, but if you feel the surgeon is exaggerating, ask why.

The Surgery

I had to interview a lot of doctors and do a lot of reading to understand exactly what every cosmetic surgery procedure is (they all have ridiculously long formal names, but I will use the more common terms). I can give you a capsule review of each procedure, the pain involved (frankly, much of this made me sick to even think about), your down time, and the cost. The costs I give are national averages (costs may be higher or lower in your area) from 1994, the most recent year for which information was available, and are for the surgeon's fee only. Operating-room and anesthesia costs are extra. You still need to grill your surgeon for a more complete description of each procedure. He or she should take you through everything step-by-step, from the moment you arrive for surgery to your care up to a year afterward. Surgeons develop new techniques all the time, so don't be surprised if my descriptions of the procedures and recovery differ slightly from your surgeon's.

You should also discuss with your doctor what remedies he/she will offer if something does go wrong. Many surgeons will redo the procedure for free (although you'll still pay for the operating-room and anesthetic costs). Learn this information ahead of time.

I am especially grateful to two surgeons who provided guidance in describing each procedure and making sure I got the facts right. They are Steven J. Pearlman, M.D., F.A.C.S., associate director of the Department of Head and Neck Surgery at St. Luke's Roosevelt Hospital Center and assistant professor of Otolaryngology at Columbia University College of Physicians and Surgeons, both in New York City, and Thomas Romo III, M.D., director of Facial and Plastic Surgery at Lenox Hill Hospital and director of Facial Plastic and Reconstructive Surgery at New York Eye and Ear Infirmary, both in New York City.

Types of Anesthesia

Your surgeon will decide, with you, which type of anesthesia to use during your surgery. General anesthesia requires the presence of an anesthesiologist, which will mean another doctor's fee for you.

LOCAL: You are awake and area of surgery is numbed by an injection.

LOCAL WITH SEDATION: You are sedated with a pill or an intravenous drug such as Valium. You are not completely asleep but you will feel sleepy and feel no pain. Frequently, and more safely, given by an anesthesiologist.

GENERAL ANESTHESIA: You are put to sleep by an intravenous drug or gas. You will feel no pain during surgery, but will take longer to recover because the anesthesia lingers in your body for about a week.

Face- and Neck-Lift

WHAT IT IS: A face- and neck-lift will tighten loose, sagging skin and make some wrinkles disappear. It will make you look good for your age, but not necessarily ten years younger.

THE PROCEDURE: The surgeon will make an incision starting in front of the ear, around the bottom, up the back of the ear into the hairline. He will then lift the facial skin and muscles and pull snugly (but not tightly) toward incision. He will suture first the muscle and then the skin, trimming any excess skin.

If a neck-lift is also being done—it's a part of almost all face-lifts unless not needed—the surgeon will make a small incision under your chin, suction out fat, and tighten the neck muscle.

TYPE OF ANESTHESIA: Local with sedation

SURGERY TIME: 3 to 4 hours

RECOVERY TIME: You will be swollen and bruised for about two weeks, but will have very little pain other than pressure and tightness in the face. (Occasionally, the surgeon will have to put little drains at suture site to drain excess blood from surgery. If so, you will have a little pain until they are removed in two days.)

Depending on the type of stitches or staples your surgeon uses, they will be removed five to fourteen days after surgery.

You will have noticeable scars around your ears for a while. These can usually be covered by your hair. It may take six months to a year before scars fade to a thin line. You may be one of those people who heal poorly. If so, your scars may be redder and deeper than you expected. If you are really unhappy, ask your surgeon if minor surgery will diminish scars.

COST: Face-lift, $4,293; neck-lift (if done with face-lift), $1,000

Upper Eyelid Surgery

WHAT IT IS: This surgery removes loose skin, fat, and stretched muscle over eyes. You will have a more noticeable eyelid and a younger appearance. This is not a brow-lift and won't remove crow's feet.

THE PROCEDURE: The surgeon will make an incision along your natural eyelid crease and remove excess skin. He will then remove excess fat. Small stitches will close the incision.

TYPE OF ANESTHESIA: Local with light sedation

SURGERY TIME: 1 to 1½ hours

RECOVERY TIME: Your lids will be swollen and sore for about five days. Stitches can be removed two to five days after surgery. Eyes will be sensitive to light and dust for about two weeks (contacts shouldn't be worn for about two weeks). Your eyelids may remain numb for a while—six weeks is common. There will be a faint scar in the crease of your lid; severity depends on your healing process.

COST: $1,545

Lower Eyelid Surgery

WHAT IT IS: This surgery will remove bags and puffy areas beneath the eye. It will not eliminate wrinkles because the skin here cannot be pulled tight (that would just pull your eye down). It will get rid of some wrinkles, but don't expect too much. (Wrinkles can be removed if the surgeon does laser resurfacing.)

THE PROCEDURE: The surgeon will make an incision just below your eye, pull skin back, and remove the fat that is causing your bumps or puffiness. He will then close the incision and if there is extra skin will snip that off and stitch the wound closed. If you are only having fat removed from under the eye, a completely hidden incision can be made inside your eyelid. This results in no external scarring.

TYPE OF ANESTHESIA: Local with sedation

SURGERY TIME: About 1 to 2 hours

RECOVERY TIME: You will have some soreness and bruising under your eyes for about two weeks. The bruising will slowly fall down your face (due to gravity) and disappear. Stitches will be removed a few days after surgery (unless incision was made inside lid, then there are no stitches). You can wear mascara on lower lashes to cover scarring after about a week (ask your surgeon). Eventually, the scar will fade to a very faint and unnoticeable line under lower lashes.

COST: $1,594

Brow-Lift

WHAT IT IS: This procedure will smooth out the skin on your forehead and between brows. It will not completely eliminate all wrinkles (and you wouldn't want it to; you'd look expressionless), but will leave you with a smooth and more youthful-looking forehead. It will also lift eyebrows to eliminate sagging. This part of the surgery may work so well that you will not need an eyelid-lift if you were planning one. If you are having both surgeries done at once, ask your surgeon to do brow-lift first and then decide if you need the eyelid-lift.

THE PROCEDURE: Some surgeons use the older procedure: The surgeon will make an incision from ear to ear over the top of your head, behind the hairline. He will then lift the skin and cut the muscles and fat underneath. He will also cut into the muscle between your brows to flatten the indentation between eyes. He will then pull the skin up over your forehead and stitch, cutting off excess skin. A newer, less-invasive option is using an endoscope (sort of like a telescope that can see under the skin). The results look more natural and the procedure can be done with only four tiny incisions.

TYPE OF ANESTHESIA: Local with sedation

SURGERY TIME: Between 1 and 2 hours

RECOVERY TIME: You will have a throbbing headache for a few days, which can be treated with pain medication. You will have bruising and swelling that will gradually move down your face. This will last about two weeks. You will also have some numbness and itching along incision line (endoscopic surgery will cause less of this). Your stitches will be removed in about six days. You will see no permanent scars because they are covered by the hairline (although hair may thin temporarily).

COST: $2,130

Nose Surgery

WHAT IT IS: Nose surgery can do many things. Surgery can be done to remove a small bump or the entire nose can be rebuilt, including reshaping the nostrils or removing a big tip. Each procedure is slightly different and recovery varies. Ask your surgeon for the specifics of what you want done. Nose surgery will not give you someone else's nose, it will give you a new version of your own nose.

If you had a nose job as a teenager and you are not happy with it, it can be redone. If the nose has collapsed or drooped, there are new procedures using silicone implants to rebuild the nose. Since this procedure is new, make sure your surgeon is well-trained in performing it.

THE PROCEDURE: The surgeon will work on your nose from the inside, leaving no visible scars (unless you are having nostrils trimmed, in which case you will have small scars in creases next to nostrils). To trim a bump the surgeon will remove the excess cartilage by shaving it down. To thin the nose on the sides the surgeon will have to chisel bones down. If you are only having the end of your nose reshaped, the surgeon will go in through nostrils and remove tissue from the tip to diminish size.

TYPE OF ANESTHESIA: Local with sedation or general

SURGERY TIME: About 1 to 2 hours

RECOVERY TIME: The surgeon will pack your nose with gauze and cover it with a plaster bandage. You will have to breathe out of your mouth for a few days, which can cause dry mouth and cracked lips. Your face will be swollen and your nose will hurt. Bruising will occur over the next few days (mostly under eyes) and will take about two weeks to go away. Swelling may take longer to subside. You may see the difference in your nose immediately, but it takes up to a full year before the final effects are in place.

COST: $2,879

Chin Surgery

WHAT IT IS: Surgery on the chin is mostly done to create a stronger jawline and improve the look of your profile. This is done by inserting an implant. Chin surgery is also done to reshape or reduce the size of the chin. This is done by shaving and reshaping the bone.

THE PROCEDURE: Implant: Your surgeon can make an incision either under your chin or inside your lower lip. He will lift tissue away from bone to make a space for the implant. He will then insert the implant and stitch it in. Then he stitches the incision closed.

Reshaping: The surgeon makes an incision inside lower lip and lifts the tissue away from the bone to expose the chin. The surgeon uses an electric saw to chisel away parts of bone. To keep your new chin shape in place, the surgeon will attach metal wires or a metal plate. Muscles and mouth tissue are then stitched.

TYPE OF ANESTHESIA: Local with sedation or general

SURGERY TIME: About 1 hour, slightly longer to reshape bone

RECOVERY TIME: There should be very little pain after implant surgery and mild pain after a reshaping. Your chin will be numb for awhile, about two to six weeks, and will be swollen for about two weeks and may be bruised. Some swelling will remain for a while. Give it six months before you assess results.

COST: Implant, $1,216; reshaping, $1,984

Cheek Implant

WHAT IT IS: Cheek-implant surgery will give your face more shape and definition.

THE PROCEDURE: Incision is made inside the upper lip, leaving no outside scarring. The surgeon then lifts the cheek tissue off the bone and inserts the implant in-between. The incision is then stitched closed.

TYPE OF ANESTHESIA: Local with sedation

SURGERY TIME: About an hour

RECOVERY TIME: You will not have much pain after cheek-implant surgery. You will have some swelling and light bruising for about two weeks. It may take about six weeks before your cheeks lose the numb feeling and six months for all of the swelling (you will hardly notice this) to disappear.

COST: $1,800

Breast Enlargement

WHAT IT IS: This surgery increases the size of the breast by the use of implants. Most surgeons now use saline implants, which have proven to be safer than silicone.

THE PROCEDURE: The surgeon will make an incision underneath or on the side of your breast. If implant is going between the muscle and the breast, the surgeon will cut all of the fibers that attach the breast to the muscle to create a pocket for the implant. If the implant is going under muscle, the surgeon will cut through muscle, then remove the muscle from the ribs and slip the implant in underneath it. He will then close the incision.

TYPE OF ANESTHESIA: Local with sedation or general if implant is placed beneath the muscle

SURGERY TIME: About 1 to 2 hours

RECOVERY TIME: You will feel a little pain and swelling in your breasts right after surgery. Your breasts will look larger than they will eventually be, because of swelling. This should go away in about six weeks. You will need to wear a bra day and night for a few weeks to support your new breasts. Stitches will be removed in about ten days. Scarring will eventually diminish to a faint line.

COST: $2,417

Breast-Lift

WHAT IT IS: This surgery will lift drooping breast and reposition nipple. The size of your breasts will stay the same, the shape will change.

THE PROCEDURE: There are two parts to this surgery. First the surgeon will make an incision underneath the breast and from the bottom to nipple. He will pull down excess skin, trim, and stitch. Next he will remove the nipple (but not completely), leaving important nerves attached. This is a newer procedure called superior pedicle surgery. It results in leaving you with sensation in your nipples and less chance of failure when moving the nipple. He will move the nipple into its new position and stitch.

TYPE OF ANESTHESIA: Local with sedation or general

SURGERY TIME: About 1 to 2 hours

RECOVERY TIME: You will have pain and swelling in your breasts after surgery. Soreness should disappear during the first week, swelling in about six weeks. Depending on the type of stitches used, they will be removed within five days to two weeks. You will have scars, but their severity depends on how your body heals. Don't expect scars to really fade for about a year.

COST: $3,148

Breast Reduction

WHAT IT IS: This surgery will give you smaller breasts. Most women undergo breast reduction because the size of their breasts causes back and shoulder pain or because they feel self-conscious about being so large.

THE PROCEDURE: The surgeon prepares the new nipple site then cuts around nipple, leaving blood vessels and nerves intact. He will then cut into breast to remove excess tissue to achieve your desired size. He will then stitch nipple in place and close vertical and horizontal incisions.

TYPE OF ANESTHESIA: General

SURGERY TIME: Between 2 and 4 hours

RECOVERY TIME: You will really hurt for a few days after this surgery. Most pain can be controlled by medication, which is why you will probably stay in the hospital at least overnight. You will need oral pain medication for about two weeks. Your breasts will be bruised for about a week and swollen for up to six. You will have to wear a bra day and night and not be able to shower for about a week. Stitches are removed in five to fifteen days. You will always have some scarring, but the severity depends on how you heal.

COST: $4,741

Tummy Tuck

WHAT IT IS: This surgery removes excess skin and fat, and tightens loose stomach muscles. A "mini-tuck" only cuts off excess skin (if you've lost a lot of weight and have folds across your tummy, this may be all you need).

THE PROCEDURE: This is pretty major surgery and you may need to stay in the hospital overnight or for a few days if your surgeon wants you to. The surgeon starts by making an incision around your navel and suctioning out fat (see Liposuction for process). He will then make an incision just above your pubic bone and stitch your stomach muscles tight. The skin is then pulled tight and excess trimmed. The surgeon may now do additional suctioning of fat around sides of tummy and then stitch incision closed.

TYPE OF ANESTHESIA: General

SURGERY TIME: Between 2 and 4 hours

RECOVERY TIME: You will have pain after surgery and be given pain medication in the hospital. You will also be fed intravenously for about two days to prevent vomiting, which will pull on stitches inside. You'll also have a catheter so you won't have to get up and urinate. You may feel pain for about two weeks as muscles heal. You will be bruised and swollen for a few weeks also. Stitches may be removed in stages: some after a week, others after two weeks.

COST: $3,776

Arm-Lift

WHAT IT IS: This surgery will trim skin and suction excess fat to correct sagging upper arms.

THE PROCEDURE: The surgeon will make an incision down the inside, underneath section of your arm. He will then remove excess fat and skin and sew incision closed.

TYPE OF ANESTHESIA: Local with sedation

SURGERY TIME: About 2 hours

RECOVERY TIME: Your arms will be a little sore, swollen, and bruised. Pain can be controlled by oral pain medication. Stitches will be removed in about five days. You will probably always have some scarring—the skin here is tender—but since it will be on the inside of your arm it will not be that visible.

COST: $2,471

Buttock-Lift

WHAT IT IS: This surgery will lift and tighten your bottom.

THE PROCEDURE: The surgeon will make an incision in the crease between your bottom and your thigh. He will then remove excess skin and a thick layer of fat from the buttocks. He will then pull the skin tight and stitch closed.

TYPE OF ANESTHESIA: General

SURGERY TIME: Between 2 and 3 hours

RECOVERY TIME: These days this may be an outpatient operation, but your surgeon may also recommend that you stay overnight in the hospital to control pain. You will be sore, bruised, and swollen. Your legs may swell for about a week after surgery. Most stitches will be removed in about a week; some may stay in for two weeks. Scarring should be hidden by the natural crease below your bottom, but if you look closely you will be able to see it.

COST: $3,171

Liposuction

WHAT IT IS: The surgeon will use a cannula—a sticklike instrument—to suck fat from just about anywhere in your body. The most common areas are the hips, thighs, and buttocks. This surgery is not for the obese, but more to reshape individual body parts.

THE PROCEDURE: The surgeon makes a tiny incision in the area to be suctioned and then pushes the cannula through. He has to move the tube back and forth to gather fat (it looks like he's pumping). When he's done suctioning he will close the incision.

TYPE OF ANESTHESIA: Local with sedation or general

SURGERY TIME: About 1 to 2 hours per site

RECOVERY TIME: You will have a little pain, bruising, and swelling around the site for a few days. You will have to wear a surgical support for about two weeks. You will see results after swelling subsides (about two weeks). Stitches are removed in about a week and you will have only a tiny scar at each site.

COST: $1,639

After researching and writing this chapter, I still don't know if I will ever have cosmetic surgery. It seems less scary to me now though. Maybe when I'm sixty I *will* have a face-lift. . . . Oh, I don't know . . . maybe not.

Okay, This Is It . . .

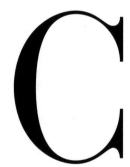ongratulations! To you and to me.
To me because I actually wrote this book. To you because
you read it. Wow! Together we have accomplished a lot. I'll
bet you look great. And you know what . . . it didn't hurt a
bit, did it? (Maybe getting rid of your favorite skirt from
the seventies stung for a minute, but you did it). How do
you feel? Different? Funny? Silly? Strange? Or do you feel
pretty? If you're just starting out on this journey you will
feel prettier and prettier and prettier every day. All you have to do is look into the
faces of the people who love you and you'll know.

You probably didn't take every piece of advice I gave you. That's okay. I know
you're taking what you need to be a better you. That's what it's all about. That's why
I wrote this book. I wanted all of you to know that you can learn about fashion and
style, and that you never have to feel inadequate or awkward or afraid. You can feel
great about yourself.

Now that you know the rules, you'll make fewer fashion mistakes. You'll still
make a few—I do—but that's okay because you'll recognize them sooner. You'll see
a great green jacket and then remember that green is not one of your four colors;
you'll come across an old purple mascara and toss it, remembering that it doesn't fit

the new you. You'll start to pay attention to the details of dressing well and sooner or later it will all become second nature.

Where do you go from here? Well, after you get the fundamentals of style down pat, that's when you can really begin to have fun. You can then buy a trendy skirt because you know how to integrate it into your wardrobe and you'll know when to stop wearing it because the trend is over. You can even start to build a second wardrobe in another basic color. The world is open to you.

In the end, everything I've told you here is to help you bring out the best of you. Let the world see what a terrific person you are. Pour yourself a glass of champagne and toast yourself. You've done it, girl. You've made the changes you wanted to make. You've done it from the inside out and from the outside in. You know what? I'm proud of you.